Hyperthyroidism - Recent Updates

Edited by Volkan Gelen,
Abdulsamed Kükürt and Emin Şengül

Published in London, United Kingdom

Hyperthyroidism - Recent Updates
http://dx.doi.org/10.5772/intechopen.100994
Edited by Volkan Gelen, Abdulsamed Kükürt and Emin Şengül

Contributors
Fida Hussain, Muhammad Adil, Mehmood Hussain, Javaid Ahmad Bhat, Shoiab Mohd Patto, Pooran Sharma, Mohammad Hayat Bhat, Shahnaz Ahmad Mir, Charles Bitamazire Businge, Vulikhaya Mpumlwana, Constance Nontsikelelo Gubu-Ntaba, Nandipha Mizpa Sotobe-Mbana, Chukwuma Ogbonna Ekpebegh, Martha Mayer, Volkan Gelen, Emin Şengül, Abdulsamed Kükürt, Stefan Schopf, Elias Karakas, Mustafa Cesur, Irmak Sayin Alan, Swarnkumar Reddy, Hari Krishnan Krishnamurthy, Vasanth Jayaraman, Karenah E. Rajasekaran, Tianhao Wang, Kang Bei, Karthik Krishna, John J. Rajasekaran

First published in London, United Kingdom, 2023 by IntechOpen
IntechOpen is the global imprint of INTECHOPEN LIMITED, registered in England and Wales, registration number: 11086078, 5 Princes Gate Court, London, SW7 2QJ, United Kingdom

British Library Cataloguing-in-Publication Data
A catalogue record for this book is available from the British Library

Additional hard and PDF copies can be obtained from orders@intechopen.com

Hyperthyroidism - Recent Updates
Edited by Volkan Gelen, Abdulsamed Kükürt and Emin Şengül
p. cm.
Print ISBN 978-1-83969-981-8
Online ISBN 978-1-83969-982-5
eBook (PDF) ISBN 978-1-83969-983-2

Meet the editors

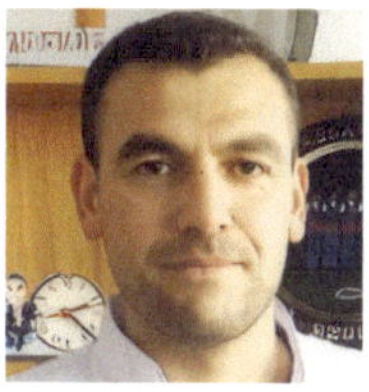

Dr. Volkan Gelen is a physiology specialist who received his veterinary degree from Kafkas University, Turkey, in 2011. From 2011 to 2015, he worked as an assistant in the Department of Physiology, Faculty of Veterinary Medicine, Atatürk University, Turkey. In 2016, he joined Kafkas University as an assistant professor where he has been engaged in various academic activities. Dr. Gelen has sixty journal articles and twenty poster presentations to his credit. His research interests include physiology, the endocrine system, cancer, diabetes, cardiovascular diseases, and isolated organ bath system studies.

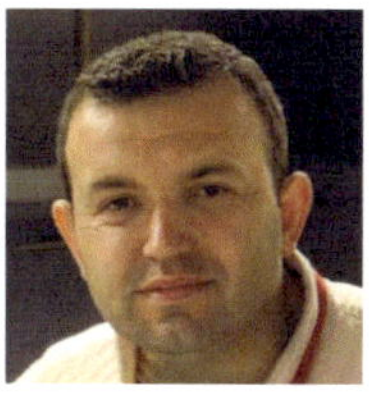

Dr. Abdulsamed Kükürt graduated from Uludağ University, Turkey. In 2019, he obtained a Ph.D. in Biochemistry from the Institute of Health Sciences, Kafkas University, Turkey, where he is currently an assistant professor in the Department of Biochemistry. He has published twenty-eight research articles in academic journals, eleven book chapters, and thirty-seven papers. Dr. Kükürt has participated in ten academic projects and is a reviewer for many academic journals.

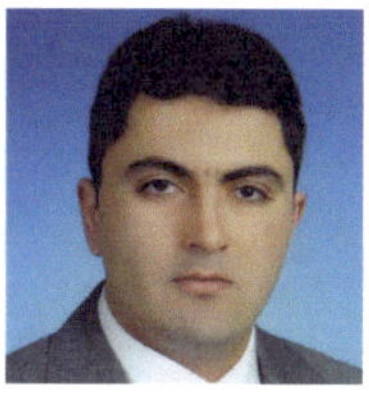

Dr. Emin Şengül is a physiology specialist who received his veterinary degree from Atatürk University, Turkey, in 2008. In 2014, he became an assistant professor at the same university. He has published sixty-two journal articles and given twenty poster presentations at scientific congresses. His research interests include physiology, the endocrine system, cancer, diabetes, gastric ulcer, neurotoxicity, testicular toxicity, nephrotoxicity, cardiovascular diseases, and isolated organ bath system studies.

Contents

Preface

Hyperthyroidism involves physiological, biological, and clinical factors that cause hypermetabolism due to the excessive elevation of thyroid hormones in the blood and the surrounding tissues under the influence of high levels of hormones. There is a general acceleration in metabolism. The term 'thyrotoxicosis' is sometimes used to describe this syndrome. Symptoms include irritability, nervousness, excessive sweating, increased blood pressure and breathing, tachycardia, shortness of breath, diarrhea, goiter, exophthalmos, and skin changes. Graves' disease is a very common autoimmune disease. Antithyroid drugs, lithium carbonate, radioactive iodine, and dexamethasone are used in the treatment of hyperthyroidism. Thyrotoxicosis is characterized by hypermetabolism and hyperactivity syndrome, in which serum concentrations of T4, T3, or both are increased. Diseases that cause hyperthyroidism can originate from the thyroid gland, as well as from pituitary or non-pituitary causes. Hyperthyroidism is categorized into three groups: primary, secondary, and subclinical hyperthyroidism. This book provides comprehensive and important information on the secretion and functions of thyroid hormones, as well as the causes, types, symptoms, associated diseases, and treatments of hyperthyroidism.

Volkan Gelen,
Faculty of Veterinary Medicine,
Department of Physiology,
Kafkas University,
Kars, Turkey

Abdulsamed Kükürt,
Faculty of Veterinary Medicine,
Deparment of Biochemistry,
Kafkas University,
Kars, Turkey

Emin Şengül,
Faculty of Veterinary Medicine,
Department of Physiology,
Atatürk University,
Erzurum, Turkey

Section 1

Introduction

Chapter 1

Introductory Chapter: The Relationship between Hyperthyroidism and Oxidative Stress-Mediated Cell Damage

Volkan Gelen and Abdulsamed Kükürt

1. Introduction

Oxidative stress describes the pathological condition that occurs as a result of the reaction of reactive oxygen species with various biomolecules in the organism [1]. It may occur as a result of the increase of free oxygen radicals in the body and the synthesis of nitric oxide [2, 3]. The free radicals formed combine with the DNA, carbohydrates, lipids, and proteins in the cell and cause the cell structure to deteriorate [4–6]. In addition, lipid peroxidation occurs as a result of the reaction of lipids in the cell membrane with free radicals [7]. MDA, the intermediate product of this reaction, is formed [8]. MDA formation is directly proportional to the cell membrane's damage and irreversible damage [9]. Free radicals cause DNA double helix cleavage and nucleic acid base exchange, thus making DNA ready for mutation [10, 11]. Again, free radicals cause protein oxidation [12]. As a result of this reaction, the function of the proteins is impaired and the enzymatic reactions in which the proteins take part, the transport systems, and the functions of the receptors are impaired [13]. In addition, reactive oxygens oxidize monosaccharides to form oxoaldehydes, which cross-link with DNA and RNA [14]. This leads to cancer and aging. In addition, reactive oxygen species cause the destruction of immune system cells, thus weakening the immune system [15]. There are some antioxidant-effective enzymes as a protective system in the organism against this damage [16]. They protect the cell from oxidative stress by scavenging free oxygen radicals or reducing their effects [17]. Antioxidants are divided into two groups, enzymatic and non-enzymatic. While antioxidants such as superoxide dismutase (SOD), catalase, glutathione peroxidase (GSH-Px), peroxidase, and glutathione reductase (GR) are classified as enzymatic, GSH, vitamin C, urate, bilirubin, albumin, ceruloplasmin, transferrin, and lactoferrin are classified as non-enzymatic [18–20]. Thyroid hormones increase the metabolic activity of tissues in most living organisms [21, 22]. Thyroid hormones show their effect on energy metabolism, oxygen consumption, and some mitochondrial functions including oxidative phosphorylation, and by increasing mitochondrial respiration by making many changes in the activity and number of some mitochondrial respiratory chain components [23, 24]. With the effectiveness of thyroid hormones, superoxide formation in the mitochondrial electron transport system increases [25]. As a result of this increase, oxidative stress and cell damage occur [26]. The metabolic effects of thyroid

 IntechOpen

hormones are well known, but the effects of thyroid hormone deficiency and excess on lipid peroxidation and antioxidant system have not been clearly demonstrated [27, 28]. In this section, we aimed to explain the mechanism of the relationship between hyperthyroidism and oxidative stress-mediated cell damage.

2. Hyperthyroidism and oxidative stress

Hyperthyroidism is defined as excessive secretion of thyroid hormones. Thyroid hormones increase basal metabolism and thus oxidative metabolism by inducing specific mitochondrial enzymes [29]. Therefore, hyperthyroidism accelerates the formation of free oxygen radicals and causes evenings in the antioxidant defense system [30] (**Figure 1**). As a result of increased free radical formation in patients with hyperthyroidism, changes in the concentrations of other related molecules (antioxidants, lipid peroxides) are expected [31]. It has been stated that there may be a relationship between the physiopathology of this disease and free radicals and antioxidants [32]. Defects in the antioxidant enzyme system can lead to the accumulation of reactive oxygen derivatives [33]. ROS targets protein oligosaccharides and alters their biological functions [34]. Due to oxidative stress, the extracellular matrix glycosaminoglycan structure is destroyed [35]. Hydrogen peroxide, formed due to the catalysis of superoxide ions by superoxide dismutase, is used as a substrate for thyroid hormone synthesis by thyroid peroxidase [36]. In a study, it was reported that the GSH level was significantly reduced in patients with hyperthyroidism [37]. Again, some studies determined that MDA levels increased in various tissues of patients with hyperthyroidism, and SOD activity decreased [38]. Thyroid hormones cause a hypermetabolic state by changing the activity and number of mitochondrial respiratory chain components and increasing the mitochondrial respiratory rate. The accelerated mitochondrial electron transport also increases the formation of superoxide, and in this way, the formation of many reactive species occurs [39]. As a result of oxidative stress and impaired antioxidant defense mechanism, cell membranes and organelles are damaged.

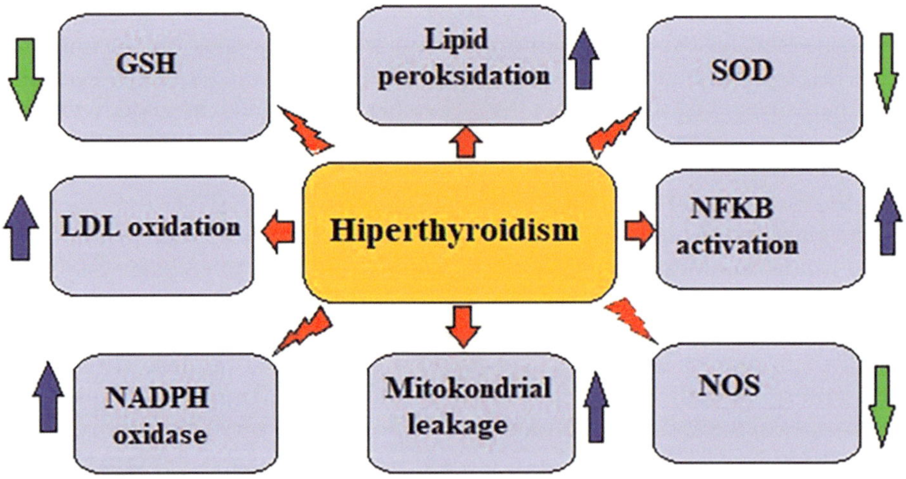

Figure 1.
Hyperthyroidism and oxidative stress.

3. Conclusion

As a result, hyperthyroidism is a pathological condition that occurs as a result of excessive secretion of thyroid hormone. In the case of hyperthyroidism, the increased thyroid hormone level causes an increase in the metabolic activity of the tissues. Particularly with the effectiveness of thyroid hormones, superoxide formation in the mitochondrial electron transport system increases. Increasing metabolic activity not only triggers the production of free oxygen radicals but also disrupts the antioxidant defense mechanism. In this case, increasing free oxygen radicals react with lipids, proteins, and carbohydrates in the cell membrane and disrupt their structure and activities. In this case, disruptions occur in reactions such as substance transport, enzymatic activity, and cell communication in the cell. Thus, hyperthyroidism causes oxidative stress-mediated cell damage.

Author details

Volkan Gelen[1*] and Abdulsamed Kükürt[2]

1 Faculty of Veterinary Medicine, Department of Physiology, Kafkas University, Kars, Türkiye

2 Faculty of Veterinary Medicine, Department of Biochemistry, Kafkas University, Kars, Türkiye

*Address all correspondence to: gelen_volkan@hotmail.com

References

[1] Jakubczyk K, Dec K, Kałduńska J, Kawczuga D, Kochman J, Janda K. Reactive oxygen species—Sources, functions, oxidative damage. Polski Merkuriusz Lekarski: Organ Polskiego Towarzystwa Lekarskiego. 2020;**48**:124-127

[2] Tan BL, Norhaizan ME, Liew W-P-P. Nutrients and oxidative stress: Friend or foe? Oxidative Medicine and Cellular Longevity. 2018;**9719584**

[3] Yang S, Lian G. ROS and diseases: Role in metabolism and energy supply. Molecular and Cellular Biochemistry. 2020;**467**:1-12

[4] Gelen V, Şengül E, Yıldırım S, Senturk E, Tekin S, Kükürt A. The protective effects of hesperidin and curcumin on 5-fluorouracil–induced nephrotoxicity in mice. Environmental Science and Pollution Research. 2021;**28**:47046-47055. DOI: 10.1007/s11356-021-13969-5

[5] Yun HR, Jo YH, Kim J, Shin Y, Kim SS, Choi TG. Roles of autophagy in oxidative stress. International Journal of Molecular Sciences. 2020;**21**:3289

[6] Sies H. Oxidative stress: A concept in redox biology and medicine. Redox Biology. 2015;**4**:180-183

[7] Gelen V, Şengül E. Antioxidant, antiinflammatory and antiapoptotic effects of naringin on cardiac damage induced by cisplatin. Indian Journal of Traditional Knowledge. 2020;**19**:459-465

[8] Kara A, Gedikli S, Sengul E, Gelen V, Ozkanlar S. Oxidative stress and autophagy. In: Ahmad R, editor. Free Radicals and Diseases. London: IntechOpen; 2016. pp. 69-86. DOI: 10.5772/64569

[9] Sengul E, Gelen V, Yildirim S, Cinar İ, Aksu EH. Effects of naringin on oxidative stress, inflammation, some reproductive parameters, and apoptosis in acrylamide-induced testis toxicity in rat. Environmental Toxicology. 2023 Mar;**38**(4):798-808

[10] Gu Y, Han J, Jiang C, Zhang Y. Biomarkers, oxidative stress and autophagy in skin aging. Ageing Research Reviews. 2020;**59**:101036

[11] Vostrikova SM, Grinev AB, Gogvadze VG. Reactive oxygen species and antioxidants in carcinogenesis and tumor therapy. Biochemistry (Moscow). 2020;**85**:1254-1266

[12] Kükürt A, Gelen V, Başer ÖF, Deveci HA, Karapehlivan M. Thiols: Role in oxidative stress-related disorders. In: Atukeren P, editor. Accenting Lipid Peroxidation. London: IntechOpen; 2021. pp. 27-47. DOI: 10.5772/intechopen.96682

[13] Jakubczyk K, Kałduńska J, Dec K, Kawczuga D, Janda K. Antioxidant properties of small-molecule non-enzymatic compounds. Polski Merkuriusz Lekarski: Organ Polskiego Towarzystwa Lekarskiego. 2020;**48**:128-132

[14] Kowalska K, Brodowski J, Pokorska-Niewiada K, Szczuko M. The change in the content of nutrients in diets eliminating products of animal origin in comparison to a regular diet from the area of Middle-Eastern Europe. Nutrients. 2020;**12**:2986

[15] Gelen V, Yıldırım S, Şengül E, Çınar A, Çelebi F, Küçükkalem M, et al. Naringin attenuates oxidative stress, inflammation, apoptosis, and oxidative DNA damage in acrylamide-induced nephrotoxicity in rats. Asian Pacific

Journal of Tropical Biomedicine. 2022;**12**(5):223-232

[16] Sies H, Jones DP. Reactive oxygen species (ros) as pleiotropic physiological signalling agents. Nature Reviews. Molecular Cell Biology. 2020;**21**:363-383

[17] Gelen V, Kükürt A, Şengül E, Devecı HA. Leptin and its role in oxidative stress and apoptosis: An overview. In: Role of Obesity in Human Health and Disease. [Working Title]. London, UK: IntechOpen; 2021. DOI: 10.5772/intechopen.101237

[18] Kim Y-M, Kim S-J, Tatsunami R, Yamamura H, Fukai T, Ushio-Fukai M. ROS-induced ROS release orchestrated by Nox4, Nox2, and mitochondria in VEGF signaling and angiogenesis. American Journal of Physiology. Cell Physiology. 2017;**312**:C749-C764

[19] Aldosari S, Awad M, Harrington EO, Sellke FW, Abid MR. Subcellular reactive oxygen species (ROS) in cardiovascular pathophysiology. Antioxidants Basel Switzerland. 2018;7:14

[20] Irazabal MV, Torres VE. Reactive oxygen species and redox signaling in chronic kidney disease. Cell. 2020;**9**:1342

[21] Garmendia Madariaga A, Santos Palacios S, Guillén-Grima F, Galofré JC. The incidence and prevalence of thyroid dysfunction in Europe: A meta-analysis. The Journal of Clinical Endocrinology and Metabolism. 2014;**99**:923-931

[22] Canaris GJ, Manowitz NR, Mayor G, Ridgway EC. The Colorado thyroid disease prevalence study. Archives of Internal Medicine. 2000;**160**:526-534

[23] Kasagi K, Takahashi N, Inoue G, Honda T, Kawachi Y, Izumi Y. Thyroid function in Japanese adults as assessed by a general health checkup system in relation with thyroid-related antibodies and other clinical parameters. Thyroid. 2009;**19**:937-944

[24] Empson M, Flood V, Ma G, Eastman CJ, Mitchell P. Prevalence of thyroid disease in an older Australian population. Internal Medicine Journal. 2007;**37**:448-455

[25] Rostami R, Aghasi MR, Mohammadi A, Nourooz-Zadeh J. Enhanced oxidative stress in Hashimoto's thyroiditis: Interrelationships to biomarkers of thyroid function. Clinical Biochemistry. 2013;**46**:308-312

[26] Ameziane El Hassani R, Buffet C, Leboulleux S, Dupuy C. Oxidative stress in thyroid carcinomas: Biological and clinical significance. Endocrine-Related Cancer. 2019;**26**:R131-R143

[27] Fahim YA, Sharaf NE, Hasani IW, Ragab EA, Abdelhakim HK. Assessment of thyroid function and oxidative stress state in foundry workers exposed to lead. Journal of Health and Pollution. 2020;**10**:200903

[28] Lassoued S, Mseddi M, Mnif F, Abid M, Guermazi F, Masmoudi H, et al. A comparative study of the oxidative profile in Graves' disease, Hashimoto's thyroiditis, and papillary thyroid cancer. Biological Trace Element Research. 2010;**138**:107-115

[29] Eleutherio ECA, Magalhães RSS, de Araújo Brasil A, Neto JRM, de Holanda Paranhos L. More than just an antioxidant. Archives of Biochemistry and Biophysics. 2021;**15**(697):108701

[30] Sepasi Tehrani H, Moosavi-Movahedi AA. Catalase and its mysteries. Progress in Biophysics and Molecular Biology. 2018;**140**:5-12

[31] Couto N, Wood J, Barber J. The role of glutathione reductase and related enzymes on cellular redox homoeostasis

network. Free Radical Biology & Medicine. 2016;**95**:27-42

[32] Metere A, Frezzotti F, Graves CE, Vergine M, De Luca A, Pietraforte D, et al. A possible role for selenoprotein glutathione peroxidase (GPx1) and thioredoxin reductases (TrxR1) in thyroid cancer: Our experience in thyroid surgery. Cancer Cell International. 2018;**18**:7

[33] Torun AN, Kulaksizoglu S, Kulaksizoglu M, Pamuk BO, Isbilen E, Tutuncu NB. Serum total antioxidant status and lipid peroxidation marker malondialdehyde levels in overt and subclinical hypothyroidism. Clinical Endocrinology. 2009;**70**:469-474

[34] Erdamar H, Cimen B, Gülcemal H, Saraymen R, Yerer B, Demirci H. Increased lipid peroxidation and impaired enzymatic antioxidant defense mechanism in thyroid tissue with multinodular goiter and papillary carcinoma. Clinical Biochemistry. 2010;**43**:650-654

[35] Loomis SJ, Chen Y, Sacks DB, Christenson ES, Christenson RH, Rebholz CM, et al. Cross-sectional analysis of AGE-CML, SRAGE, and EsRAGE with diabetes and cardiometabolic risk factors in a community-based cohort. Clinical Chemistry. 2017;**63**:980-989

[36] Ruggeri RM, Giovinazzo S, Barbalace MC, Cristani M, Alibrandi A, Vicchio TM, et al. Influence of dietary habits on oxidative stress markers in Hashimoto's thyroiditis. Thyroid. 2021;**31**:96-105

[37] Kasai H. Analysis of a form of oxidative DNA damage, 8-hydroxy-20-deoxyguanosine, as a marker of cellular oxidative stress during carcinogenesis. Mutation Research/Reviews in Mutation Research. 1997;**387**:147-163

[38] Rovcanin BR, Gopcevic KR, Kekic DL, Zivaljevic VR, Diklic AD, Paunovic IR. Papillary thyroid carcinoma: A malignant tumor with increased antioxidant defense capacity. The Tohoku Journal of Experimental Medicine. 2016;**240**:101-111

[39] Ates I, Arikan MF, Altay M, Yilmaz FM, Yilmaz N, Berker D, et al. The effect of oxidative stress on the progression of Hashimoto's thyroiditis. Archives of Physiology and Biochemistry. 2018;**124**:351-356

Section 2

Effects of Thyroid Hormones on the Organism

Chapter 2

Thyroid Hormones (T3 and T4) and Their Effects on the Cardiovascular System

Volkan Gelen, Emin Şengül and Abdulsamed Kükürt

Abstract

Thyroid hormones (thyroxine, triiodothyronine) have a metabolic effect on many tissues and systems in the organism. Therefore, in case of deficiency or excess of these hormones, some problems arise. The decrease in the effect of these hormones in the peripheral target tissue is called hypothyroidism, the picture characterized by excessive secretion of the thyroid gland or being of non-thyroid origin is called hyperthyroidism. Thyroid hormone disorders are common in the world. Knowing the functions of thyroid hormones, which have such important effects on the organism, is important in developing treatment options for the problems to be encountered. In the literature reviews, it has been stated that thyroid hormones have some effects such as heart rate, myocyte contraction, blood pressure, plasma lipid level, and thrombogenesis. In line with this information, the presented section has tried to explain how the mechanism of the effects of thyroid hormones on the cardiovascular system.

Keywords: TSH, T4, T3, hyperlipidemia, thrombogenesis, blood pressure

1. Introduction

The thyroid gland, which is the largest of the endocrine glands and is located in the right and left lobes on both sides of the end of the larynx and the beginning of the trachea, is histologically composed of many spherical follicles. The space in the middle of the follicle surrounded by a single layer of epithelial cells is filled with a substance called colloid. The main substance of the colloid is a large glycoprotein, namely thyroglobulin, which also contains the gland hormones like thyroxine (T4) and triiodothyronine (T3) [1]. These hormones are secreted as a result of stimulation of the thyroid gland by the thyroid-stimulating hormone (TSH) released from the pituitary [2]. The thyroid gland shows its effects on the target tissue through these two hormones. Of these hormones, T3 has a much stronger effect than T4. T4 is converted to T3 by monodeiodinization in the periphery [3]. T3 exerts its effects at nuclear and non-nuclear levels. Its effects at the nuclear level are through the regulation of gene expression [4]. These hormones released from the thyroid gland affect metabolic processes in almost all tissues [5–8]. Insufficient or excessive secretion of these hormones causes many problems in the organism. As a result of various studies, it has been reported that the effects of thyroid hormones on the cardiovascular system are very important and prominent [9]. It shows this effect in two ways: direct and indirect. In line with this information, in the presented section, the synthesis of thyroid hormones, their mechanisms of action, and their effects on the cardiovascular system and the mechanism of these effects will be discussed.

2. Thyroid hormones

Thyroid hormones are thyroxine (T4) and 3,5,3′ triiodothyronine (T3) and these hormones are released into the blood by being released from the thyroid gland. These hormones are very important for normal growth and development and the normal functioning of metabolism. In addition to these hormones, the calcitonin hormone, which is involved in Ca metabolism, is also released from parafollicular C cells in the thyroid gland [7].

2.1 Synthesis of thyroid hormones

The release of thyroid hormones from the thyroid gland is under the control of the TRH hormone released from the hypothalamus. TRH released from the hypothalamus stimulates the pituitary gland to release TSH. TSH released from the pituitary stimulates the thyroid gland and ensures the release of hormones from here [10]. Thyroid hormones are attached to the thyroglobulin molecule in the thyroid gland. These hormones, which are stored in the thyroid gland, are given to the blood circulation when needed. In general, the synthesis of thyroid hormones consists of 5 stages. These stages are as follows, in order: (1) uptake of iodine ion into the gland, (2) oxidation of iodine and iodination of the tyrosyl groups of thyroglobulin, (3) coupling of iodotyrosine residues with ether bonds (coupling) to form iodothyronines, (4) proteolysis of thyroglobulin and thyroxine (T4). Release of T3) into the blood, (5) conversion of thyroxine to triiodothyronine in both the thyroid gland and peripheral tissues [7, 11]. When the T3 and T4 hormones released into the blood under the control of these hormones reach a certain level, they stop the release by having a feedback effect on the hypothalamus and pituitary gland [12].

Although T3, one of the thyroid hormones, is released from the thyroid gland, the source of 80% of the circulating T3 is T3, which is formed as a result of the metabolism of T4 in peripheral tissues. The enzyme that provides the transformation in question is iodothyronine-5′-deiodinase. The place where the transformation takes place the most is the liver. The source of T3 used in many peripheral tissues is the hormone released as a result of this transformation. Unlike these tissues, locally synthesized T3 is used in the brain and pituitary gland. When thyroid hormones are released into the blood, they are transported in the blood by noncovalent binding to plasma proteins. At the beginning of these transporters is thyroxine-binding globulin (TBG). T4 binds to this binder with high affinity, whereas T3 has less affinity. T4 also binds to transthyretin (transthyretin: thyroxine-binding prealbumin) (**Figure 1**) [7, 13, 14].

2.2 Mechanism of action of thyroid hormones

Considering the mechanisms of action of thyroid hormones in the cell, T3 is clamped to high-affinity nuclear receptors on the cell surface, which then binds to a specific DNA sequence (thyroid hormone response element: TRE) in the promoter/regulatory regions of specific genes. In this way, T3 modulates gene transcription and ultimately protein synthesis. The binding of T3 to the receptor can activate gene

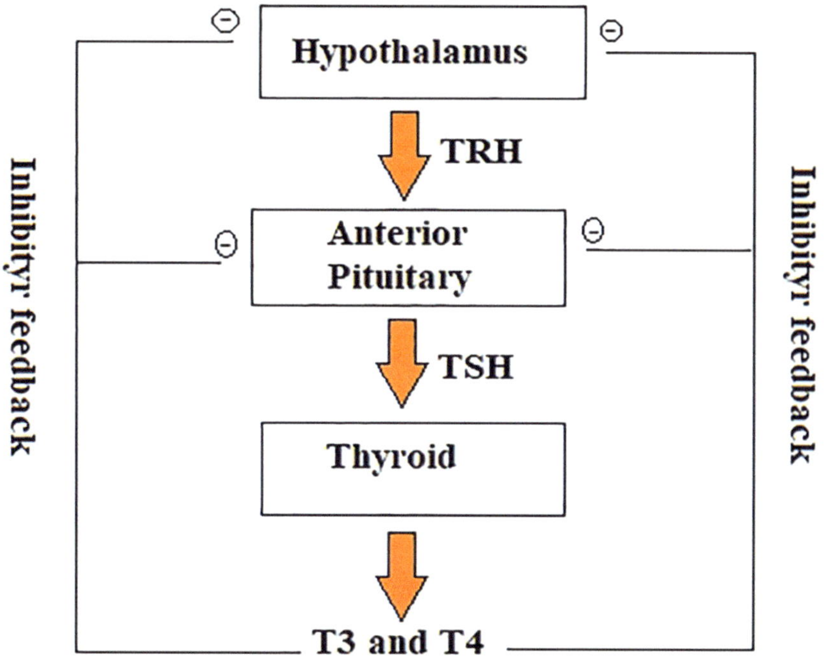

Figure 1.
Control of synthesis of thyroid hormones [7].

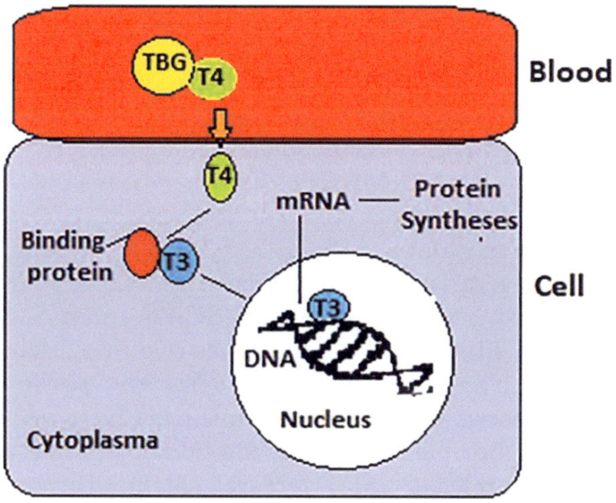

Figure 2.
Mechanism of action of thyroid hormones on target cell [7].

transcription by removing suppression. The interaction of hormones with their receptors can cause direct stimulating or suppressive effects. Although T4 also binds to the aforementioned receptors, it shows less affinity than T3. In addition, despite its ability to bind to nuclear receptors, T4 does not have a gene transcription-modifying effect [15]. Therefore, T4 appears to be more of a prohormone, and the effects of TH are considered to be mainly through T3 [16]. TH also exerts some of its effects on receptors in mitochondria. These hormones increase the oxidative metabolism of mitochondria, oxygen consumption, and ATP formation in some cell types (**Figure 2**) [17, 18].

3. Effects of thyroid hormones on the cardiovascular system

Thyroid hormone (TH) receptors (TRs) are located in the myocardium and vascular endothelium, so changes in circulating TH concentration have an effect on cardiac and vascular functions. In patients with hypo- or hyperthyroidism, cardiovascular (CV) and hematological manifestations occur. Minor changes in TH concentration may have an adverse effect on the CV system, and subclinical thyroid dysfunction may result in a 20–80% increase in the risk of vascular morbidity and mortality [19, 20, 21].

3.1 Thyroid hormone and heart rate

Heart rate is an important mechanism in the regulation of the cardiac output, which specifically determines the cardiac ejection rate. It also affects systolic and diastolic functions [22]. Considering the relationship between thyroid hormone and heart rate, studies have shown that thyroid hormone has a consistent positive chronotropic effect and causes resting sinus tachycardia [23].

3.2 Effect of thyroid hormones on cardiac myocytes

The genomic effects of TH are mediated by TH nuclear receptors in the cell. Protein receptors bind to T3 with more than 10-fold greater affinity than T4 [24]. In mammals, there are two isoforms of these receptor proteins, a and b (TRa and TRB). TRa and TRB activate the expression of positively regulated genes in the presence of T3 and suppress expression in their absence. It has been determined that the TRa1 isoform plays an important role in the regulation of cardiac genes. It contains myosin heavy chain an (a-MHC) and myosin heavy chain b (b-MHC) as contractile apparatus of cardiac myocytes. The fast myosin a-MHC and the slow myosin b-MHC are positively and negatively regulated by T3. Cardiac contractility is further regulated by several important cardiac proteins, including sarcoplasmic reticulum calcium adenosine triphosphatase (SERCA2) and its inhibitory counterpart, phospholamban (PLB). SERCA2 functions to pump calcium (Ca2+) ions back into the sarcoplasmic reticulum during the relaxation phase of myofilament contraction. T3 positively regulates SERCA2 while negatively regulating PLB. SERCA2 and PLB are responsible for calcium ion influx into the sarcoplasmic reticulum and subsequent release [25]. Decreased calcium turnover in cardiac myocytes has been reported in hypothyroidism with impaired diastolic function. Other important cardiac genes regulated by TH include those encoding TR proteins themselves, voltage-gated potassium ion (K+) channels, and sodium/calcium ion (Naþ/Ca2+) exchanger (NCX1).TH (both T4 and T3) exerts non-genomic effects on cardiac myocytes and vessels. Non-genomic effects usually occur at the receptor-independent plasma membrane and regulate ion transporter activity [26]. These combined mechanisms at the atrial myocyte level are partly responsible for the heart rate-enhancing effect of T3 [27].

3.3 Effect of thyroid hormones on vascular

When the effects of TH on the vessels are examined, it is seen that the effect occurs at the vascular smooth muscle and endothelial cell levels. TH acts through ion channel activation (Na+, K+, Ca2+) and regulation of specific signal transduction pathways. It also activates the phosphatidylinositol 3-kinase and serine/threonine protein kinase pathways, resulting in nitric oxide production from the endothelium. Thus, it causes a decrease in systemic vascular resistance through its effects on vascular smooth muscle cells [28]. Some studies have shown that TH regulates endothelial nitric oxide production and vascular tone, and patients with hypothyroidism exhibit impaired endothelial function, which is improved by TH replacement therapy [29–31]. In addition, T3 may produce a vasodilator effect within hours after the application in patients undergoing coronary artery bypass grafting [32]. Similar effects are observed when patients with chronic heart failure are treated with intravenous T3 [33]. T3, therefore, has the unique pharmacological properties of an indicator acting primarily on diastolic dysfunction. TH does not have vasodilator effects in the pulmonary vasculature or systemic vasculature [34].

3.4 Cardioprotective effect of thyroid hormones

THs are involved in cardioprotection through the activation of cytoprotective mechanisms, stimulation of cell growth, neoangiogenesis, and metabolic adaptation. Recent experimental studies using the ischemia/reperfusion rat model have shown that TH has multiple protective effects, particularly on mitochondria. TH is a regulator of the tumor suppressor p53, which is activated during acute myocardial infarction (AMI) and enhances the mitochondrial apoptosis pathway [35]. This promotes p53 accumulation and, therefore, increases mitochondrial dysfunction and BCL-2-like protein 4 activation, leading to the prolongation of myocardial cell loss [36]. T3 treatment counteracts the reduction in miR-30a levels, thereby limiting p53 activation and the cascade that leads to mitochondrial damage and cell death in the AMI border region [37]. In addition, T3 treatment preserves the expression of hypoxia-inducible factor 1-alpha, whose protective effect against reperfusion injury is mediated by inhibiting the mitochondrial opening of permeability passage pores [38]. THs have an antiapoptotic effect on myocytes through activation of phosphatidylinositol 3-kinase/serine/threonine protein kinase and protein kinase C signaling cascades, expression, phosphorylation and translocation of heat shock proteins 70 and 27, and suppression of p38 mitogen [39].

3.5 Thyroid hormones and blood pressure

Considering the effects of hyperthyroidism on blood pressure, it causes hyperdynamic circulation, which causes an increase in cardiac contractility and thus increases heart rate, again with increased preload and decreased systemic vascular resistance (SVR). As a result, cardiac output increases. Although hyperthyroidism can increase systolic blood pressure, the net effect depends on the balance between increased cardiac output and decreased SVR [40, 41]. Endothelium-dependent vasodilation is lower in patients with severe hypothyroidism and SCH [42] and improves with levothyroxine therapy, as is the pulse-wave rate [43, 44], a surrogate measure of arterial stiffness. Various factors possibly contribute to arterial stiffness and endothelial dysfunction in SCH and hypothyroidism, including hyperlipidemia and a proinflammatory state [45–47]. Both hyperlipidemia and thyroid antibodies are thought to reduce endothelial nitric oxide synthase expression and thus impair vasodilation.

3.6 Thyroid hormones and hyperlipidemia

Hyperthyroidism lowers cholesterol levels, which reverses when euthyroidism is reached. Hypothyroidism is associated with a small but significant increase in lipid parameters [38], particularly the elevation of low-density lipoproteins (LDLs) [48]. Hypothyroidism is associated with increased oxidation of LDL, which promotes atherogenesis and improves with treatment [49, 50]. Lipoprotein(a), a stronger marker of atherogenesis, is also increased in overt hypothyroidism and decreased with TH replacement [51, 52]. In hypothyroidism, hyperlipidemia results from a decrease in LDL receptors, resulting in decreased cholesterol clearance from the liver and decreased cholesterol-clearing activity of cholesterol 7α-hydroxylase activated by TH [48]. In addition, thyroid hormones stimulate lipoprotein lipase (LPL), which catabolizes TG-rich lipoproteins, and hepatic lipase (HL), which hydrolyses HDL2 to HDL3 and contributes to the conversion of medium-density lipoproteins (IDL) to LDL. Another effect of T3 is the up-regulation of apolipoprotein AV (ApoAV), which plays an important role in TG regulation. In studies, this situation has been associated with increased ApoAV levels and decreased TG levels.

3.7 Thyroid hormones and thrombogenesis

Overt and SHyper have been associated with increased markers of thrombogenesis (fibrinogen and factor X levels) [53, 54]. Hyperthyroid patients may have higher von Willebrand antigen levels than euthyroid patients, resulting in increased platelet plug formation, decreasing after treatment [55]. Interestingly, a study comparing patients with moderate and severe hypothyroidism with euthyroid controls found that patients with moderate hypothyroidism had reduced fibrinolytic activity and were more susceptible to clot formation, while patients with severe hypothyroidism had increased fibrinolysis and lower tissue plasminogen activator antigen [56]. The effects of TH on platelet function are unclear [55].

4. Conclusion

In conclusion, this section presents the importance of thyroid hormones for the organism and the synthesis steps of these hormones, their transport in the blood, and their effects on the cardiovascular system. The mechanisms of these effects are discussed by reviewing the current literature. This study aims to present current literature information to researchers who will work on this subject.

Author details

Volkan Gelen[1]*, Emin Şengül[2] and Abdulsamed Kükürt[3]

1 Faculty of Veterinary Medicine, Department of Physiology, Kafkas University, Kars, Turkey

2 Faculty of Veterinary Medicine, Department of Physiology, Atatürk University, Erzurum, Turkey

3 Faculty of Veterinary Medicine, Department of Biochemistry, Kafkas University, Kars, Turkey

*Address all correspondence to: gelen_volkan@hotmail.com

References

[1] Emirzeoğlu M, ve Sancak, R. Tiroit bezi anatomisi. Journal of Experimental and Clinical Medicine. 2012;**29**(4S):273-275

[2] Bostancı N. Paratiroid Hastalıkları. Bozak Matbaası: İstanbul; 1979. pp. 199-248

[3] Cooper DS. Hyperthyroidism. The Lancet. 2003;**362**:459-468

[4] Parry C. Palpitation of the heart in connection with enlargement of the thyroid. Disease Heart. 1825;**2**:111-165

[5] Osman F, Gammage MD, Franklyn JA. Thyroid disease and its treatment: Short-term and long-term cardiovascular consequences. Current Opinion in Pharmacology. 2001;**1**:626-631

[6] Keçeci T, ve Kocabatmaz M. Hipotiroidizmin kan üre azotu, total protein, glikoz ve total kolesterol düzeyleri üzerindeki etkisi. Veteriner Bilimler Dergisi 1994;**10**(1-2):134-138

[7] Hall JE. Guyton and Hall Textbook of Medical Physiology Elsevier Health Sciences. USA: Elsevıer; 2010

[8] Davison K, Potter G, Evans J, Greene L, Hargis P, Corn C, et al. Growth, nutrient utilization, radiographic bone characteristics and postprandial thyroid hormone concentrations in weanling horses fed added dietary fat. Journal of Equine Veterinary Science. 1991;**11**(2):119-125

[9] Toft AD, Boon NA. Thyroid disease and the heart. Heart. 2000;**84**:455-460

[10] Frates MC, Benson CB, Charboneau JW, Cibas ES, Clark OH, Coleman BG, et al. Management of thyroid nodules detected at US: Society of radiologists in ultrasound consensus conference statement. Ultrasound Quarterly. 2006;**22**(4):231-238

[11] Gardner DG, Shoback D, ve Greenspan FS. Greenspan's Basic & Clinical Endocrinology. China: McGraw-Hill Medical; 2007

[12] Gharib H, Papini E, Paschke R, Duick D, Valcavi R, Hegedüs L, et al. American association of clinical endocrinologists, associazione medici endocrinologi, and european thyroid association medical guidelines for clinical practice for the diagnosis and management of thyroid nodules. Endocrine Practice. 2010;**16**(Suppl. 1):1-43

[13] Goudreau E, Comtois R, Bayardelle P, Beauregard H, ve Larochelle D. Capnocytophaga ochracea and group F beta-hemolytic streptococcus suppurative thyroiditis. The Journal of Otolaryngology. 1986;**15**(1):59-61

[14] Vasudevan DM, Sreekumari S. Thyroid hormones. In: Textbook of Biochemistry. 4th ed. New Delhi: Jaypee; 2004

[15] White BA, Porterfield SP. The thyroid gland. In: White BA, Porterfield SP, editors. Endocrine and Reproductive Physiology. 4th ed. Philadelphia: Elsevier; 2013. pp. 129-147

[16] Salvatore D, Simonides WS, Dentice M, Zavacki AM, Larsen PR. Thyroid hormones and skeletal muscle — New insights and potential implications. Nature Reviews. Endocrinology. 2014;**10**(4):206-214

[17] Oppenheimer JH, Schwartz HL, Lane JT, Thompson MP. Functional

relationship of thyroid hormoneinduced lipogenesis, lipolysis and thermogenesis in the rat. The Journal of Clinical Investigation. 1991;**87**(1):125-132

[18] Weintraub M, Grosskopf I, Trostanesky Y, Charach G, Rubinstein A, Stern N. Thyroxine replacement therapy enhances clearance of chylomicron remnants in patients with hypothyroidism. The Journal of Clinical Endocrinology and Metabolism. 1999;**84**(7):2532-2536

[19] Biondi B, Cooper DS. The clinical significance of subclinical thyroid dysfunction. Endocrine Reviews. 2008;**29**:76-131

[20] Jabbar A, Razvi S. Thyroid disease and vascular risk. Clinical Medicine (London, England). 2014;**14**(Suppl. 6): s29-s32

[21] Jabbar A, Pingitore A, Pearce SH, Zaman A, Iervasi G, Razvi S. Thyroid hormones and cardiovascular disease. Nature Reviews. Cardiology. 2017;**14**:39-55

[22] Nordyke RA, Gilbert FI Jr, Harada AS. Graves' disease. Influence of age on clinical findings. Archives of Internal Medicine. 1988;**148**:626-631

[23] von Olshausen K, Bischoff S, Kahaly G, Mohr-Kahaly S, Erbel R, Beyer J, et al. Cardiac arrhythmias and heart rate in hyperthyroidism. The American Journal of Cardiology. 1989;**63**:930-933

[24] Sandler B, Webb P, Apriletti JW, et al. Thyroxine-thyroid hormone receptor interactions. The Journal of Biological Chemistry. 2004;**279**:55801-55808

[25] Dillmann W. Cardiac hypertrophy and thyroid hormone signaling. Heart Failure Reviews. 2010;**15**:125-132

[26] Davis PJ, Goglia F, Leonard JL. Nongenomic actions of thyroid hormone. Nature Reviews. Endocrinology. 2016;**12**:111-121

[27] Klein I. Chapter 81: Endocrine disorders and cardiovascular disease. In: Braunwald's Heart Disease. 10th ed. Philadelphia, Pennsylvania: Elsevier; 2014. pp. 1793-1808

[28] Carrillo-Sepúlveda MA, Ceravolo GS, Fortes ZB, et al. Thyroid hormone stimulates NO production via activation of the PI3K/Akt pathway in vascular myocytes. Cardiovascular Research. 2010;**85**:560-570

[29] Papaioannou GI, Lagasse M, Mather JF, Thompson PD. Treating hypothyroidism improves endothelial function. Metabolism. 2004;**53**:278-279

[30] Taddei S, Caraccio N, Virdis A, et al. Impaired endothelium-dependent vasodilatation in subclinical hypothyroidism: Beneficial effect of levothyroxine therapy. The Journal of Clinical Endocrinology and Metabolism. 2003;**88**:3731-3737

[31] Razvi S, Ingoe L, Keeka G, Oates C, McMillan C, Weaver JU. The beneficial effect of l-thyroxine on cardiovascular risk factors, endothelial function, and quality of life in subclinical hypothyroidism: Randomized, crossover trial. The Journal of Clinical Endocrinology and Metabolism. 2007;**92**:1715-1723

[32] Klemperer JD, Klein I, Gomez M, et al. Thyroid hormone treatment after coronary-artery bypass surgery. The New England Journal of Medicine. 1995;**333**:1522-1527

[33] Pingitore A, Galli E, Barison A, et al. Acute effects of triiodothyronine (T3) replacement therapy in patients with

chronic heart failure and lowT3 syndrome: A randomized, placebo-controlled study. The Journal of Clinical Endocrinology and Metabolism. 2008;**93**:1351-1358

[34] Marvisi M, Zambrelli P, Brianti M, Civardi G, Lampugnani R, Delsignore R. Pulmonary hypertension is frequent in hyperthyroidism and normalizes after therapy. European Journal of Internal Medicine. 2006;**17**:267-271

[35] de Castro AL, Fernandes RO, Ortiz VD, Campos C, Bonetto JH, Fernandes TR, et al. Thyroid hormones improve cardiac function and decrease expression of pro-apoptotic proteins in the heart of rats 14 days after infarction. Apoptosis. Feb 2016;**21**(2):184-194

[36] Li J, Donath S, Li Y, Qin D, Prabhakar BS, Li P. miR-30 regulates mitochondrial fission through targeting p53 and the dynamin-related protein-1 pathway. PLoS Genetics. 2010;**6**:e1000795

[37] Forini F, Kusmic C, Nicolini G, et al. Triiodothyronine prevents cardiac ischemia/reperfusion mitochondrial impairment and cell loss by regulating miR30a/p53 axis. Endocrinology. 2014;**155**:4581-4590

[38] Pantos C, Mourouzis I, Dimopoulos A, et al. Enhanced tolerance of the rat myocardium to ischemia and reperfusion injury early after acute myocardial infarction. Basic Research in Cardiology. 2007;**102**:327-333

[39] Pantos C, Mourouzis I, Saranteas T, et al. Thyroid hormone improves postischaemic recovery of function while limiting apoptosis: A new therapeutic approach to support hemodynamics in the setting of ischaemia-reperfusion? Basic Research in Cardiology. 2009;**104**:69-77

[40] Danzi S, Klein I. Thyroid hormone and blood pressure regulation. Current Hypertension Reports. 2003;**5**:513-520

[41] Ching GW, Franklyn JA, Stallard TJ, Daykin J, Sheppard MC, Gammage MD. Cardiac hypertrophy as a result of long-term thyroxine therapy and thyrotoxicosis. Heart. 1996;**75**:363-368

[42] Lekakis J, Papamichael C, Alevizaki M, et al. Flow-mediated, endothelium-dependent vasodilation is impaired in subjects with hypothyroidism, borderline hypothyroidism, and high-normal serum thyrotropin (TSH) values. Thyroid. 1997;**7**:411-414

[43] Dernellis J, Panaretou M. Effects of thyroid replacement therapy on arterial blood pressure in patients with hypertension and hypothyroidism. American Heart Journal. 2002;**143**:718-724

[44] Obuobie K, Smith J, Evans LM, John R, Davies JS, Lazarus JH. Increased central arterial stiffness in hypothyroidism. The Journal of Clinical Endocrinology and Metabolism. 2002;**87**:4662-4666

[45] Taddei S, Caraccio N, Virdis A, et al. Low-grade systemic inflammation causes endothelial dysfunction in patients with Hashimoto's thyroiditis. The Journal of Clinical Endocrinology and Metabolism. 2006;**91**:5076-5082

[46] Türemen EE, Çetinarslan B, Şahin T, Cantürk Z, Tarkun I. Endothelial dysfunction and low grade chronic inflammation in subclinical hypothyroidism due to autoimmune thyroiditis. Endocrine Journal. 2011;**58**:349-354

[47] Marazuela M, Sánchez-Madrid F, Acevedo A, Larrañaga E, de Landázuri MO. Expression of vascular adhesion molecules on human endothelia in autoimmune thyroid disorders.

Clinical and Experimental Immunology. 1995;**102**:328-334

[48] Duntas LH. Thyroid disease and lipids. Thyroid. 2002;**12**:287-293

[49] Diekman T, Demacker PN, Kastelein JJ, Stalenhoef AF, Wiersinga WM. Increased oxidizability of low-density lipoproteins in hypothyroidism. The Journal of Clinical Endocrinology and Metabolism. 1998;**83**:1752-1755

[50] Costantini F, Pierdomenico SD, De Cesare D, et al. Effect of thyroid function on LDL oxidation. Arteriosclerosis, Thrombosis, and Vascular Biology. 1998;**18**:732-737

[51] Tzotzas T, Krassas GE, Konstantinidis T, Bougoulia M. Changes in lipoprotein(a) levels in overt and subclinical hypothyroidism before and during treatment. Thyroid. 2000;**10**:803-808

[52] Martinez-Triguero ML, Hernández-Mijares A, Nguyen TT, et al. Effect of thyroid hormone replacement on lipoprotein(a), lipids, and apolipoproteins in subjects with hypothyroidism. Mayo Clinic Proceedings. 1998;**73**:837-841

[53] Dörr M, Robinson DM, Wallaschofski H, et al. Low serum thyrotropin is associated with high plasma fibrinogen. The Journal of Clinical Endocrinology and Metabolism. 2006;**91**:530-534

[54] Erem C. Blood coagulation, fibrinolytic activity and lipid profile in subclinical thyroid disease: Subclinical hyperthyroidism increases plasma factor X activity. Clinical Endocrinology. 2006;**64**:323-329

[55] Homoncik M, Gessl A, Ferlitsch A, Jilma B, Vierhapper H. Altered platelet plug formation in hyperthyroidism and hypothyroidism. The Journal of Clinical Endocrinology and Metabolism. 2007;**92**:3006-3012

[56] Chadarevian R, Bruckert E, Leenhardt L, Giral P, Ankri A, Turpin G. Components of the fibrinolytic system are differently altered in moderate and severe hypothyroidism. The Journal of Clinical Endocrinology and Metabolism. 2001;**86**:732-737

Section 3

Hyperthyroidism Treatment Options

Chapter 3

Radioactive Iodine Therapy for Hyperthyroidism

Fida Hussain, Muhammad Adil and Mehmood Hussain

Abstract

Hyperthyroidism is one of the most commonly encountered endocrine disorder with potentially devastating health consequences. Radioactive iodine has been used for the treatment of hyperthyroidism since 1940s. It is now widely accepted as safe, cost-effective and reliable treatment option with 50–90% cure rate in first year after therapy. With long-term follow-up hypothyroidism is inevitable especially in Grave's disease which can activate orbitopathy in predisposed individuals. Early and timely management of hypothyroidism is associated with better therapeutic outcomes. There is very little evidence of cardiovascular and cancer related mortality risk after radioactive iodine therapy. However, it is said that these risks appear to be thyroid hormone driven above all other factors.

Keywords: Grave's disease, hyperthyroidism, radioactive iodine, thyrotoxicosis, toxic nodular goiter

1. Introduction

Thyroid dysfunctions are commonly encountered in clinical practice affecting a considerable portion of population. However, incidence and pattern of thyroid disease vary significantly depending upon age, gender, ethnicity and geographical distribution [1]. Global prevalence of hyperthyroidism varies from 0.2 to 1.3% in different studies [2]. Thyroid dysfunction has important ramifications on health outcome especially in older population like cardiovascular, metabolism, bone and mental health. Undiagnosed and untreated hyperthyroidism causes drastic clinical complications for patients as well as health care delivery system in term of economic burden. Hence early diagnosis and prompt treatment are indispensable to reduce mortality and associated costs [3].

Radioactive Iodine (RAI) represents as an effective treatment modality for hyperthyroidism, especially in cases who do not respond to medical therapy. RAI therapy is in practice for the last 80 years. It was first used for therapeutic purpose in 1941 by Dr. Saul Hertz [4]. Over the time its therapeutic efficacy was evaluated and evolved, by 1990 it becomes preferred treatment option for Grave's disease in US. Although, previously it was reserved for patients who had a relapse after failed medical treatment. New practice guidelines of National Institute for Health and Care Excellence (NICE) recommends RAI as first line treatment option in cases of Grave's disease [5].

This chapter focuses on the role of radioactive iodine in hyperthyroidism and other related therapeutic aspects with a background knowledge of pathophysiology of thyroid gland.

2. Thyroid hormone synthesis

Thyroid hormones, L-thyroxine (tetraiodothyronine, T4) and L-triiodothyronine (T3) are the only iodine containing molecules in vertebrates with well-established biological role. Baumann was the first to report the presence of iodine in thyroid hormone in 1895 with iodine accounting for 65% of T4 and 58% of T3 weight. Iodine is an integral component and rate-limiting substrate for thyroid hormone synthesis that is provided exogenously. Ingested iodine is absorbed from small intestine as iodide into the plasma which also contains iodide released by thyroid gland and extrathyroidal deiodination of iodothyronines. This iodide is either transported in plasma and taken up by thyroid or excreted via urine.

Thyroid follicles, the structural and functional unit of thyroid are responsible for production, storage and secretion of thyroid hormones. Iodide is actively trapped into thyroid follicular cells (thyrocytes) against electrochemical gradient by sodium-iodide symporter (NIS) at basolateral membrane while efflux of iodide across apical membrane into follicular lumen is mediated by Pendrin, a potential iodide transporter. Normally, thyroid concentrates 20–50 times higher iodide as compared to plasma. Inside thyroid follicle iodide is rapidly oxidized to iodine by thyroid peroxidase (TPO) in the presence of hydrogen peroxidase generated by membrane bound NADPH-oxidase. Iodine is then covalently bound to the selected tyrosyl residues of thyroglobulin (Tg) at the apical plasma membrane-follicle lumen boundary resulting in the formation of monoiodotyrosine and diiodotyrosine (MIT, DIT), a process referred to as organification or iodination. Tg is the most abundant protein in thyroid providing polypeptide backbone for thyroid hormone synthesis and storage. Subsequently, two neighboring iodotyrosyl residues on Tg molecule are coupled in the presence of TPO to produce iodothyronine; two DIT form T4 while one DIT and one MIT form T3. Iodinated Tg is stored as colloid in follicular lumen. Upon stimulation, Tg is internalized into follicular cells by pinocytosis and digested by endosomes and lysosomes resulting in release of T4 (~80%) and T3 (~20%). Deiodination of MIT and DIT by intracellular iodotyrosine dehalogenase release iodide which is again recycled for hormone synthesis [6].

3. Regulation of thyroid hormone synthesis

Thyroid hormone synthesis is primarily governed by hypothalamic-pituitary-thyroid axis, a prime negative feedback mechanism that respond suitably to any challenge to maintain biochemical equilibrium. Hypothalamic hormone, thyrotropin releasing hormone (TRH) and thyroid stimulating hormone (TSH) or thyrotropin release by anterior pituitary stimulates thyroid hormone synthesis and secretion while thyroid hormones in turns inhibit the production and secretion of both TRH and TSH and vice versa. This complex interaction between TSH and thyroid hormones maintain serum hormone levels within narrow limit. However, this relationship is individual, dynamic and adaptive depending on many factors.

TSH almost influences every step in thyroid hormone synthesis and release via Gp/phospholipase C and cAMP cascade respectively. It stimulates thyroid cell proliferation and hormone synthesis by inducing expression of Tg, TPO, NIS and iodothyronine deiodinase type I (D1). Clinically serum TSH levels serves as sensitive biomarker for evaluation of thyroid dysfunction even at sub-clinical stage [7].

Beside this, genetics factors, endocrine mediators like estrogen and corticosteroids and local factors released by nerve endings, follicular cells and C cells are also involved in the regulation of biosynthesis of thyroid hormones. Sympathetic and immune system are also involved in regulation of thyroid hormone activity, however very less is known in this regard. Antithyroid drugs, iodide and some external compounds also influence thyroid hormone metabolism [8].

4. Hyperthyroidism and thyrotoxicosis

Hyperthyroidism is pathological condition characterized by inappropriately high levels of thyroid hormones due to its excess production and release by thyroid gland. The most common causes of hyperthyroidism are diffuse toxic goiter (Grave's disease), toxic multinodular goiter (Plummer disease) and toxic adenoma. The term thyrotoxicosis is often interchangeably used with hyperthyroidism and is characterized by elevated level of circulating thyroid hormones secondary to exogenous intake or excess release of preformed stored hormones. Thyroiditis, inflammation of thyroid gland resulting in release of stored hormones is the most frequent cause of thyrotoxicosis. Other rare causes of thyrotoxicosis are iodine-induced hyperthyroidism, post-partum thyroiditis, suppurative thyroiditis, beta human chorionic gonadotropin induced thyrotoxicosis and thyrotoxicosis factitia. Follicular thyroid carcinoma, TSH secreting pituitary adenoma and struma ovarii can also cause excess thyroid hormone levels.

4.1 Epidemiology

The prevalence of thyroid dysfunction varies by age, gender, ethnicity, geographic distribution, iodine status of the population under study and difference in diagnostic thresholds. In iodine-sufficient parts of the world, the prevalence of hyperthyroidism varies from 0.2 to 1.3% while in US it is estimated to be 1.2% (0.5% overt and 0.7% subclinical). Generally, areas with iodine deficiency have higher incidence of hyperthyroidism. For example, a 2.9% prevalence of hyperthyroidism was reported in Pescopagano, an iodin-deficient village in Italy [9]. In US Grave's disease is the most common etiology of hyperthyroidism, accounting for 60–80% cases of hyperthyroidism followed by subacute thyroiditis (15–20%), toxic multinodular goiter (10–15%) and toxic adenoma (3–5%). Females are more commonly affected by thyroid disorders as compared to male. Peak age of occurrence is second to fifth decade of life [10, 11].

4.2 Clinical presentation

Clinical manifestation is attributed to elevated thyroid hormones level causing widespread multiorgan effects. The spectrum of clinical presentation depends on age, duration and severity of illness, comorbidities and underlying cause and may range from asymptomatic in subclinical disease to life threatening in thyroid storm. Adults usually present with adrenergic symptoms like restlessness, tremors, anxiety while older patients lack sympathetic symptoms and tend to presents with less obvious symptoms like weight loss, decrease appetite, shortness of breath and cardiac manifestations like atrial fibrillation and tachycardia. Older patients are at increased risk of congestive heart failure and embolic stroke due to atrial fibrillation. Some symptoms are specific to underlying cause, like Grave's disease characterized by orbitopathy and pretibial myxedema [12, 13].

Patients with untreated or uncontrolled hyperthyroidism may land up in thyroid storm preceding severe physical or mental stress like infection or trauma. Thyroid storm is a rare life-threatening endocrine emergency. It is acute exaggerated clinical manifestation of thyrotoxic state and may cause death from multiorgan failure. Thyrotoxic patient with altered sensorium is the hallmark. Patient may present with agitation, delirium, convulsions, chorea like abnormal movements, severe hyperthermia, excessive diaphoresis, hypertension and refractory dysrhythmias. The incidence and mortality associated with thyroid storm is not precisely known. The reported incidence is 2–16% in hospitalized thyrotoxic patients with an overall mortality rate of 8–30% [12, 13].

4.3 Pathology

Grave's disease is the most frequent cause of hyperthyroidism in developed countries. It is one of most commonly encountered autoimmune disorder with peak incidence in second to fifth decade of life. Women are 5–10 times more affected. It was first described in 1834 by Robert Graves from Dublin. It is an autoimmune disorder in which antibodies against TSH receptors (TRAb) cause unopposed activation of TSH receptors triggering hormone synthesis. The usual negative feedback mechanism is not effective as the antibodies are directed against TSH receptors. This result in excessive production and release of T3 and T4, an enlarged thyroid gland and increased iodide extraction. Since TSH receptors are present in almost all tissues, extrathyroidal manifestations may be observed. Commonly observed extrathyroidal TRAb driven features are orbitopathy, pretibial myxedema and thyroid acropathy. The pathogenesis of Grave's disease is not fully understood. However, multiple risk factors are attributed to its pathogenesis. Genetic predisposition accounts for 79% while environmental factors account for 21% of the risk factors. Smoking, iodine excess, selenium and vitamin D deficiency are important environmental risk factors. Person with family history of hyperthyroidism or other autoimmune disease such as myasthenia gravis, type I diabetes mellitus are at increased risk of Grave's disease [14].

Toxic multinodular goiter (TMNG, Plummer's disease) is the second most common cause of hyperthyroidism in US after Grave's disease and most common in elderly living in iodine deficient areas. It was first described by Henry Plummer in 1913. Chronic low grade intermittent physiological or pathological stimuli can lead to diffuse or nodular enlargement of thyroid gland (goiter). Thyrotoxicosis occurs in long-standing goiter, with peak incidence in sixth or seventh decade of life. It is characterized by release of thyroid hormones by multiple autonomously functioning nodules or single autonomous nodule in thyroid gland. This functional autonomy is result of activating somatic mutations of TSH receptors genes in most of the cases (~60%). Autonomous nodules appear hots (hyperactive) on thyroid scintigraphy while non-autonomous appears as cold (hypoactive). TMNG has indolent progression with mild clinical symptoms. Clinical features are similar to thyrotoxicosis except presence of Grave's orbitopathy, dermopathy and acropathy. Compressive symptoms may also be present depending on size of gland [15].

Toxic adenoma is a benign autonomously functioning thyroid nodule with clinical and biochemical features suggestive of thyrotoxicosis. Iodine deficiency is well established risk factor in pathogenesis of adenoma besides other environmental and genetic factors. Like TMNG, activating mutations in TSH receptor genes results in toxic adenoma. The incidence is higher in women and after 50 years of age. Hyperfunctioning adenoma is usually considered as benign lesion with less than 1% chances of malignant transformation [16].

Subacute thyroiditis or de-Quervain thyroiditis is inflammation of thyroid gland that typically follow a viral infection usually upper respiratory tract infection. Recent studies have suggested that COVID-19 infection is also associated with subacute thyroiditis. This inflammatory process leads to leakage of preformed thyroid hormones into circulation and subsequently thyrotoxicosis. Patient classically presents with upper respiratory tract symptoms followed by fever, neck pain, neck swelling. Malaise, fatigue, myalgias and arthralgias are also common. Thyroid is smoothly enlarged, firm and tender on palpation. This is a self-limiting disease and usually extend over few weeks to months. About 30% of the patients undergo hypothyroidism before returning to euthyroid status due to depletion of preformed hormone stores. Approximately 10% may develop permanent hypothyroidism and require hormone replacement therapy. Subacute thyroiditis demonstrates high ESR and CRP levels and has tendency to recur [17, 18, 19].

Painless subacute thyroiditis (autoimmune or silent) is considered as a variant of Hashimoto's thyroiditis and occurs spontaneously or following pregnancy (postpartum thyroiditis). It accounts for 0.5–5% cases of hyperthyroidism. Approximately 5–20% of the patients have characteristic sequence of hyperthyroidism followed by hypothyroidism and then recovery. Thyrotoxic stage last for 2–8 weeks followed by hypothyroid stage which is usually mild or even asymptomatic and last for few weeks. It may recur in small subset of patients. About 20% of the patients develop chronic autoimmune thyroiditis and ultimately permanent hypothyroidism. Painless subacute thyroiditis is associated with specific human leukocyte antigen (HLA-DR3). Majority of the patients have elevated serum titers of antithyroid peroxidase and antithyroglobulin antibodies [18, 19].

Suppurative thyroiditis is infection of thyroid gland most commonly caused by bacteria but can also be due to fungus, mycobacterium or parasites. Acute suppurative thyroiditis is rare but life-threatening disease with estimated mortality of 3.7–9%. It is most common in immunocompromised patients. Patient usually presents with tender erythematous anterior neck swelling, fever, dysphagia and dysphonia. Acute suppurative thyroiditis can cause airway obstruction, esophageal fistula, Horner's syndrome, extension of abscess leading to mediastinitis, pericarditis, thrombophlebitis and eventually death [12].

Iodine induced hyperthyroidism (Jod-Basedow Syndrome) usually occurs in setting of underlying autonomous thyroid disease after administration of iodine, usually iodinated contrast media. Iodine provides substrate for thyroid hormone synthesis. It is common in iodine deficient areas or areas with endemic goiter. This condition is self-limiting after withdrawal of iodine with a favorable outcome. Increased iodine intake is also associated with Grave's disease [20].

There are several other but rare causes of thyrotoxicosis that deserve consideration. Beta human chorionic gonadotropin (β-hCG) can induce thyrotoxicosis by stimulating TSH receptors. Molar hydatiform pregnancies and choriocarcinoma have high level of circulating β-hCG level. Thyrotoxicosis factitia is caused by exogenous ingestion of thyroid hormones, either intentionally for therapeutic purposes or unintentionally. Patient with thyrotoxic symptoms in absence of any diagnosed thyroid disease and deranged thyroid tests should be investigated for this condition [21]. Psychiatric patients are at more risk. Some individuals use it for cosmetic reasons and to lose weight. Follicular thyroid cancer, TSH secreting pituitary adenoma and struma ovarii can also cause thyrotoxicosis in selected population [12].

4.4 Diagnosis

Diagnosis is made on the basis of history, clinical examination and relevant investigations. All patients with suspected or confirmed hyperthyroidism should be thoroughly assessed in order to formulate a treatment plan. Older patients should also be evaluated for potential cardiovascular complications.

Serum TSH and T4 estimation should be done as initial screening test. Serum TSH is more sensitive than direct thyroid hormone estimation in assessment of thyroid hormone excess. Majority of the patients (~90%) with thyrotoxicosis have raised T4 and suppressed TSH levels. However, in patients with T3 toxicosis (~5%), T3 is raised while T4 is normal. Therefore, in patients with suspected thyrotoxicosis and normal T4 levels, T3 should be done to rule out T3 toxicosis. This represents autonomously functioning thyroid nodule or initial disease stage. In patients with pituitary dependent thyrotoxicosis TSH is usually normal with raised T3 and T4. In subclinical hyperthyroidism, TSH levels are suppressed with normalized T3 and T4 while in overt hyperthyroidism T3 and T4 are elevated with suppressed TSH levels [22].

Mostly underlying etiology is suspected on the basis of clinical features like exophthalmos and goiter in Grave's disease. However, if diagnosis is not evident based on clinical and biochemical evaluation, further evaluation can be accomplished by TRAb or TSI measurements and imaging studies like radioiodine uptake (RIU) scan and thyroid ultrasonography. TRAb can confirm the diagnosis of Grave's disease with sensitivity and specificity of 97 and 99% respectively. TRAb are detected in almost all patients with Grave's disease. In USA, TRAb is only reserved for patients in whom RAIU studies are contraindicated or unavailable while in Europe TRAb is preferred over RAIU. Thyroid peroxidase (TPO) antibodies are less sensitive and specific for Grave's disease, detected in only 70–80% of patients. They are greatly influenced by environmental factors such as iodine intake [22, 23].

Ultrasound is inexpensive, non-invasive and radiation free modality to assess thyroid blood flow and suspicious thyroid nodules warranting further testing like FNAC. Doppler ultrasound examination has greatly improved accuracy specially in cases where vascularity is needed. Increased thyroid vascularity is seen in Grave's disease while decrease vascularity is indicative of destructive thyroiditis. Thyroid echogenicity assessed by ultrasonography can be used to predict remission after initiation of medications and can also identify patients who are at increased risk of recurrence after withdrawal. However, ultrasound does not precisely establish the underlying etiology of thyrotoxicosis and is reserved for cases where RAIU is contraindicated (pregnancy and breast feeding) or unavailable according to American Thyroid Association (ATA) guidelines [22, 24].

RAIU measures the percentage of radioactive iodine trapped and organified by thyroid gland after a fixed interval. It is recommended to establish the underlying etiology of thyrotoxicosis (ATA guidelines) and is preferred over TRAb estimation except in cases where RAIU is contraindicated (pregnancy and breast feeding) or unavailable. A gamma camera is used to measure the percentage of iodine uptake by gland. RAIU scan shows diffusely increased homogenous uptake in Grave's disease, focal area of increased uptake in toxic adenoma and asymmetrically irregular uptake in TMNG with multiple focal areas of increased and suppressed uptake. RAIU will be reduced or near zero in painless and subacute thyroiditis or in those with exogenous ingestion of thyroid hormones, excess iodine intake or exposure to iodinated contrast media in preceding 4–8 weeks. RAIU is also helpful in calculating therapeutic radioactive iodine dose. However, European Thyroid Association guidelines does not recommend routine use of RAIU except in cases where etiology cannot be established by laboratory and imaging studies. Technetium scintigraphy utilizes pertechnetate which is taken up by thyroid but not organified resulting in low range of uptake. The radiation exposure is less as compared to RAIU however RAIU provides more physiological information. It can also determine the underlying pathology in toxic nodular thyroid disease [22, 23, 24].

4.5 Treatment options

Treatment depends on underlying etiology and is influenced by coexisting medical condition and patient preference. There are multiple treatment strategies including antithyroid drugs (ATD), radioactive iodine (RAI) therapy and surgery along with medications for symptomatic relief.

5. Radioactive iodine therapy for hyperthyroidism

RAI-131 therapy is widely accepted and preferred treatment option for hyperthyroidism for the last eight decades. From benign nature of hyperthyroidism to malignant neoplasm and their metastasis, RAI-131 therapy has transformed patient and physician perspective towards treatment options. It was first used as therapeutic agent in 1941 for benign thyroid disease while approved by FDA in 1971 for treatment of toxic diffuse and nodular goiter, non-toxic nodular goiter and well differentiated thyroid cancer. Initially its use was only limited to elderly males with age above 50 years due to fear of associated potential risk factors at that time. However, its application has now been extended to women and children.

5.1 Historical background

Dr. E Bauman in 1895 for the first time discovered that thyroid gland contain iodide. 20 years later, it was found that gland can actively concentrate iodine. Henry Plummer, in 1923 introduce iodine as treatment adjunct for Grave's disease. Enrico in 1934 described the artificial production of radioactive isotopes including iodine which was a major breakthrough. Glenn and John in 1938 discovered radioactive iodine (RAI-131). Saul Hertz for the first to use RAI-131 in 1941 in human for the treatment of hyperthyroidism. Since then, millions of patients with benign and malignant thyroid disease have been successfully treated with RAI-131. The first patient with thyroid cancer was treated at Royal Cancer Hospital, London in 1949 [25, 26].

5.2 Properties of RAI-131

Iodine occurs naturally in stable form as I-127 with 37 known isotopes. All radioactive isotopes of iodine are produced in nuclear reactors by process of fission. I-131 is the most commonly used radioisotope of iodine with physical half-life of 8.02 days. I-131 decays to Xe-131 by emitting beta (β) particle and gamma (γ) photons. The first emission product is β-particle (90%) with end point energy of 0.606 MeV (89.7%). β-particles make I-131 a therapeutic agent as they have the propensity to ablate thyroid tissues. β-particles with these energies can only travel few millimeters ~3 mm, causing only local destruction. The second emission product is γ-photon (10%) with end point energy of 0.364 MeV (80.9%). It travels far from its source before depositing its energy with relatively little impact on thyroid tissue, hence cannot be employed for therapeutic purposes. It is however used as diagnostic tool to image thyroid [27, 28].

5.3 Pharmacokinetics of RAI-131

Pharmacokinetics of RAI-131 is similar to normal dietary iodine. After oral ingestion, sodium iodide I-131 is absorbed from small intestine into extracellular fluid. About 90% absorption occurs in first hour after ingestion. From extracellular compartment it is predominantly taken up by thyroid gland or eliminated through kidneys. NIS is responsible for active uptake of iodide in thyroid gland against electrochemical gradient. Under normal physiological condition, NIS can concentrate iodide 20–50 times of plasma concentration and this may increase up to 10 times in hyperthyroidism. Thyroid achieves its maximum uptake of iodide after 24–48 hours with 50% of maximum uptake after 5 hours. Normally thyroid has iodide clearance of about 10–50 ml/min. Iodide uptake is influenced by many factors including patient age, thyroid gland size, circulating iodide level and functional status of kidneys. After radioactive iodide uptake by thyroid, it is further oxidized to iodine and follow normal metabolism of thyroid hormone [29, 30].

NIS also mediates active RAI uptake in extrathyroidal tissues like salivary glands, lactating mammary glands, gastric mucosa, lacrimal sac and choroid plexus. However, these structures lack the system to oxidize iodide. RAI elimination from the body is mainly through renal pathway accounting for 37–75% while fecal excretion accounts for 10% of administered dose. Excretion through sweat glands is negligible [29].

5.4 Pharmaceutical preparations of RAI-131

I-131 is supplied as sodium iodide (NaI-131) in either capsule form or solution form for oral administration. Capsule are available in different activity ranging from 0.75–100 mCi. These are opaque white gelatin capsules packaged in shielded cylinders. I-131 is also available as stabilized aqueous solution in vial with activity ranging 5–150 mCi at the time of calibration. The pH of the solution is adjusted between 7.5 and 9. NaI-131 utilized in the preparation of solution at the time of calibration contains more than 99% I-131 [30].

5.5 Mode of action of RAI-131

RAI-131 emit beta particle with principal energy of 606 KeV and maximal tissue penetration of approximately 3 mm and hence can be used for therapeutic purposes. Beta irradiation causes cell death by direct and indirect damage to thyroid follicular cell's DNA predominantly through apoptosis and also necrosis. Indirect effect is mediated via release of reactive oxygen species. Another less understood mechanism is secondary immunoreactivity by released thyroid self-antigen in response to radioiodine. This immunoreactivity leads to intra-thyroidal inflammation [31].

5.6 Effective half life of RAI-131

Within a living tissue, a radionuclide decays either by physical decay (physical half-life) or biological elimination from the body (biological half-life) in an exponential pattern. Physical half-life is constant for a particular radionuclide while biological half-life is specific for patient. Overall decay of a particular radionuclide is cumulative effect of both half-lives and the half-life associated with overall decay is called effective half-life. Effective half-life is always less than isolated physical or biological half-life and is calculated as

$$1/T_{1/2}\,(\text{effective}) = 1/T_{1/2}\,(\text{physical}) + 1/T_{1/2}\,(\text{biological})$$

Effective half-life of I-131 can be estimated by measuring uptake at different time periods following administration.

5.7 Common indications

Common well-established clinical indications for RAI-131 therapy are:

- Benign thyroid disease (Grave's disease, TMNG, toxic adenoma and non-toxic nodular goiter)

- Differentiated follicular and papillary carcinoma; residual or recurrent disease after thyroidectomy, metastatic disease after near-total thyroidectomy

However, RAI-131 therapy is not only limited to these. Persistent or recurrent hyperthyroidism after partial thyroidectomy can also be treated with RAI-131. Subclinical hyperthyroidism treatment with RAI-131 has also shown promising results when underlying etiology is solitary or multiple functioning thyroid nodules or Grave's disease [32].

5.8 Treatment protocol

5.8.1 Dose calculation

RAI-131 therapy has been considered as a safe, cost-effective and durable treatment option for thyroid pathologies particularly benign thyroid disease for the last eight decades with known risk and benefits. However, optimal method of calculating RAI-131 activity to be administered to achieve therapeutic objectives is still controversial. No consensus exist on what pre-treatment measurements are required for optimal therapeutic response, balancing the risk of partial response, unnecessary radiation exposure and therapy-induced hypothyroidism. Different protocols are in use to determine the therapeutic activity in different centers. However, fixed dose method and calculating a personalized dose using either clinical scoring or scintigraphy findings are frequently used methods reported to date and studied in animals and humans.

Standard fixed dose RAI-131 therapy is simple, with early and higher cure rate and minimal remission. In this method, nuclear physician based on his personal judgment and experience prescribed a fixed dose usually ranging from 2 to 20 mCi. Different studies have been done in this regard to establish a standardized fix dose however no hard and fast rule is applied. Higher fixed dose is associated with high cure and reduced remission rate but concomitant risk of hypothyroidism. Studies show that approximately 69% patients achieve hypothyroidism at 1 year with 10 mCi RAI-131 while 75% became hypothyroid at 6 months after receiving 15 mCi [22]. However, it has been observed that same results can be obtained with different doses indicating that therapeutic outcome is not dependent only on administered activity. Studies have shown that thyroid mass and bio-kinetics also determines therapeutic outcome. Despite all these factors, European society still advocates administering fixed dose for benign thyroid disease owing to early therapeutic outcome and decrease need of retreatment [33, 34, 35].

Some studies also suggest to administer fixed dose per unit mass of thyroid gland without calculating I-131 uptake and effective half-life. It is time and cost effective and therapeutic outcomes are achieved earlier. This protocol is recommended by Society of Nuclear Medicine US and by European Association of Nuclear Medicine. Patient with small target mass will require less administered activity. However, variation in biological half-life results in over-dose, this aspect is over looked in this protocol [28].

Calculated dose protocol is based on individualized dosimetry taking into account patients anatomical and biological parameters. Idea is to calculate minimum effective dose to acquire therapeutic goals and to prevent unnecessary radiation exposure. Individual patient dosimetry is essential for determining dose–response relationship. Calculation of personalized activity to be administered depends on variables like thyroid mass, I-131 uptake values, effective half-life and dose to thyroid in grays (Gy). Some centers use fixed effective half-life of RAI-131 like 5 days for Grave's disease and 6 days for nodular goiter while other calculate on the basis of uptake values over a period of 1 week. However, calculating uptake measurements over a period of week is time-consuming, costly and inconvenient for patients. Radiation dose needed to be delivered to thyroid for therapeutic purposes following this protocol is controversial varying from low calculated dose (80 Gy) to high calculated dose (300 Gy). Low radiation dose activity is associated with less chances of hypothyroidism but increased rate of hyperthyroidism. Different algorithms are also used to calculate dose like Marinelli's formula which takes in account RAI-131 uptake and effective half-life [36, 37].

5.8.2 Patient preparation

Pre-therapy evaluation must emphasize on following:

Patient should be properly educated regarding procedure, its possible outcome, adverse events, complications, radiation safety measures they have to follow and need for long term follow-up by providing written as well as verbal information. Informed consent should be obtained prior to therapy containing all relevant information.

History including disease duration, previous treatment (ATD or RAI-131 therapy), use of iodinated contrast media or other iodine containing medications, medical therapy for other comorbid like amiodarone and urinary incontinence. Thyrostatic drugs lower radioiodine uptake and effective half-life, so they should discontinue before RAI-131 therapy. Usually, carbimazole and methimazole should be stopped 2–3 days before therapy while propylthiouracil should be discontinued 2–3 weeks prior to therapy due to more radioprotective effect because of presence of sulfhydral group. Exposure to iodine alter the timings of RAI-131 therapy. After administration of iodinated water-soluble contrast agent, therapy should be postponed for 6–8 weeks. In case of amiodarone use for underlying cardiac issue, therapy is usually not preferred because it leads to delay in excess iodine elimination for an average period of 6 months. Similarly, other iodine containing medications like lugols iodine, potassium iodide and topical iodine should be stopped 2–3 weeks before therapy [38].

Laboratory investigations including serum free T3, T4, TSH, TRAb levels.

- Recent thyroid scintigraphy and radioiodine uptake studies (< 6 months) to look for tracer uptake values and cold nodules.

- Recent ultrasound neck (< 3 months) for volume assessment and evaluation of nodules.

- Fine needle aspiration cytology of suspicious appearing nodules on ultrasound and hypo-functioning (cold) nodules on scintigraphy to exclude malignancy.

- Fasting for at least 4 hours prior to therapy and 2 hours after therapy is recommended to improve gastrointestinal absorption.

- Breast feeding and lactation are absolute contraindications for RAI-131 therapy. All women of child bearing age must be screened for pregnancy by serum or urine β-hCG levels within 24 hours of treatment. Serum β-hCG levels are more sensitive. Pregnancy test may remain negative for 7–10 days, so treating physician should discuss limitation of test in doubtful cases and delay therapy till next cycle. Post-therapy conception should be delayed for at least 6 months. This duration applies equally for males. Similarly, all potential women should be asked for breast feeding or lactation. If yes, therapy should be delayed till lactation ceases in order to minimize radiation dose to breast tissues as lactating breast can concentrate radioiodine. Usually, lactation ceases 4–6 weeks after childbirth without breast feeding or after omitting breast feeding [39].

RAI-131 is given orally as outdoor patient in facilities duly registered and authorized by regulatory bodies according to national policies. These facilities must have trained staff including nuclear physician and physicist, radiation safety procedures and equipment to handle contamination / spread and disposal of waste. If indoor therapy is recommended in some special cases, it should be done in shielded rooms.

In some cases where increased radiation dose to thyroid is needed, lithium can be used as it blocks radioiodine washout from gland without interfering with uptake. Similarly, recombinant human TSH (rhTSH) has been off label used in non-toxic MNG to maximize radiation dose to thyroid and minimize dose to reminder of the body. However, their use is still not fully documented and recommended [40].

In patients with uncontrolled urinary incontinence, proper catheterization should be done or even in-patient therapy should be considered. Literature also suggest lifelong ATD therapy in such cases if surgery is risky.

5.9 Special conditions

5.9.1 Grave's disease

As per American Thyroid Association guidelines, the aim of RAI-131 therapy is to render patient hypothyroid and it is considered as preferred treatment modality for Grave's disease in US. In Europe, ATDs are considered preferred treatment option unless patient has side effects or relapse after course of ATD, cardiac arrythmias and thyrotoxic periodic paralysis. Patients with comorbids increasing surgery risk, previously operated or irradiated, contraindications to ATD or females who are not planning pregnancy in near future (4–6 months) can be considered for therapy. Pregnancy, lactation, coexisting thyroid cancer, female planning pregnancy within

4–6 months and patients who are unable to follow radiation safety guidelines are contraindications [22, 23, 41].

Patients with overt hyperthyroidism and free T4 levels 2–3 times upper limit should be pre-treated with beta adrenergic blockers and ATD (methimazole) to prevent post-therapy worsening of symptoms. Elderly patients and those with comorbid like atrial fibrillation, heart failure, diabetes mellitus, pulmonary hypertension, renal failure and infection should get pre-therapy ATD along with optimization of their medical conditions. ATD should be stopped 3–5 days before therapy and again given 3–7 days after therapy till normalization of thyroid functions where it is tapered off. Levothyroxine substitution is started once patient become hypothyroid [42].

Grave's orbitopathy can be temporary and improves after definitive treatment of Grave's disease. In some instances, it can persist or even deteriorates after treatment. The risk of developing orbitopathy after RAI therapy is 15–30%, while its 10 and 16% after ATD and surgery respectively and it can develop any time after treatment. The deterioration of Grave's orbitopathy after RAI therapy is attributed to post-therapy hypothyroidism and increase serum level of thyroid autoantibodies. This deterioration is transient and can be managed by early initiation of thyroxin replacement and corticosteroids. Patients with pre-existing thyroid eye disease should be treated with higher radioiodine dose to achieve quick and sharper response and to avoid slow rise in autoantibodies level due to slow destruction of thyroid follicular cells. This higher dose activity along with early initiation of levothyroxine substitution can prevent worsening of disease. Euthyroid status in such patients before therapy is usually recommended. Smoking is a risk factor and predictor of therapeutic outcome and is associated with more frequent worsening and severe symptoms. A short course of low dose corticosteroids can be added with RAI therapy in non-smokers with mild active eye disease and smokers with mild or inactive eye disease. Patients with moderate to severe active thyroid eye disease should be consider for thyroid surgery or ATD. However, therapeutic efficacy of RAI in such cases needs to be evaluated [22, 23, 43].

5.9.2 Pediatric Grave's disease

Treatment options for pediatrics Grave's disease are ATD, RAI therapy and surgery. ATD are considered first-line treatment options, however incidence of relapse is very high in this age group with only 20–30% patients achieving remission after 2 years. Therefore, majority of patients need definitive treatment with either RAI ablation or surgery. The goal of RAI therapy is to achieve hypothyroidism, recommended by both ATA and ETA treatment guidelines. Usually administering high activity in single dose is recommended to prevent need of additional therapy and also minimize the risk of relapse. Low dose is associated with risk of developing nodules or malignancy at later stage in partially irradiated thyrocytes. Fixed dose (150 μCi/gm) or calculated dose protocol can be used to deliver optimal therapeutic dose. Majority of the patients (~95%) achieves hypothyroidism in 2–3 months after therapy and decrease in serum TSH level can be seen in within a week after therapy. RAI therapy should be avoided in patients with active orbitopathy [22, 43, 44].

5.9.3 Toxic nodular goiter

RAI and thyroidectomy are the two effective and safe treatment options for toxic nodular disease. The decision to select a particular treatment option is based on many factors taking into account patient preference as well. RAI is usually preferred in old age patients, patients with significant comorbids, prior surgery or irradiation to neck, small sized goiter and lack of experienced surgeon. The goal of therapy is long term alleviation of hyperthyroid state and achieve euthyroidism and volume reduction. Euthyroidism is achieved 50–60% at 3 months and 80% at 6 months after RAI therapy. Risk of hypothyroidism is very low as compared to Grave's disease. The incidence of hypothyroidism after therapy is 3% at 1 year while 64% after 20 years and more common in patients under 50 years of age.

Pretreatment with beta blockers is recommended in patients who are at risk of worsening of symptoms after therapy including elderly or those with comorbids and overt hyperthyroidism however the use of ATD before therapy needs careful monitoring and caution. ATD use before therapy can cause normal or raised TSH levels resulting in increased radiation dose to peri-nodular and contralateral thyroid tissue leading to hypothyroidism. Focal uptake in nodule with suppressed uptake in surrounding parenchyma and TSH levels is the basis of RAI treatment. Adequate radiation should be administered in single dose to achieve therapeutic goals. RAI is either given as fixed dose activity (10–20 mCi) or calculated on the basis of thyroid size and radioiodine uptake values using 150–200 μCi/gm calculated fixed dose. There is estimated 20% risk of treatment failure of TMNG and 6–18% for adenoma [22, 43, 45].

5.9.4 Non-toxic nodular goiter

Although radioiodine therapy is less commonly indicated treatment option in this group, it is still preferred in patients with recurrent goiter after surgery and comorbids which makes surgery riskier. The aim of therapy is to relive compression symptoms by volume reduction. Radioiodine uptake in non-toxic nodular goiter is usually low, sometimes even 15–20% after 24 hours of administration effecting the efficiency. This radioiodine uptake can be enhanced by low iodine diet consumption for at least 2 weeks before therapy, lithium, avoiding diuretics and recombinant human TSH (rhTSH). rhTSH can increase radioiodine uptake up to 100% without effecting half-life. However, its use is only limited in treatment of thyroid cancer. ATD can be used to increase endogenous TSH seems promising and needs further studies [46].

5.10 Follow-up

Treated patients should be regularly reviewed to assess treatment response and timely detection of radioiodine induced hypothyroidism or post-therapy immunogenic hyperthyroidism. Usually, patient respond to therapy with normalization of thyroid function test within 4–8 weeks. Hypothyroidism commonly occur between 2 and 6 months but can occur after 4 weeks after therapy. First TSH and free T4 levels should be done 4–6 weeks after therapy to detect the early effects of therapy. Subsequent visit should be done after 3 months because some patients develop severe hypothyroidism followed by yearly follow-up depending on clinical condition. Decision to start thyroxin replacement therapy depends on serum fT4 and TSH level along with clinical features. Dose should be sub-replacement level and should be titrated according to serum free T4 levels.

In cases of overt hyperthyroidism, 3–5 days after therapy ATD are usually recommended. For patients with persistent thyrotoxicosis especially Grave's disease, re-therapy is considered after 6–12 months. However, re-therapy is usually less effective due to stunning effect. In some cases, a third session may be needed if patient is still hyperthyroid. In refractory cases patient is referred for surgery [38].

5.11 Contraindications

Pregnancy and breast feeding are absolute contraindication for RAI-131 therapy. Usually, fetal thyroid tissue begins to accumulate iodine by 10–13th week of gestation. Also, radioiodine can freely cross placenta. If radioiodine is given during this period, it will damage thyroid tissue. So, all women of child bearing age should be tested for pregnancy using serum or urine β-hCG levels within 24–48 hours of therapy. Serum β-hCG level testing is more sensitive. Pregnancy test may remain negative for 7–10 days after fertilization. So, in doubtful cases patient should be counseled regarding the limitation of test and therapy be delayed till next cycle. Post-therapy conception should be delayed for 6 months to allow time for dose adjustment of thyroxin to get favorable values for pregnancy. This time also apply for male patient as well [39].

Lactating breast tissues has the ability to concentrate radioiodine maximizing radiation dose. Lactation usually ceases 4–6 weeks after child birth in the absence of breast feeding and 4–6 weeks after cessation of breast feeding. Therapy should be delayed till lactation ceases in order to minimize radiation dose to breast. Some studies suggest that breast feeding should not be resumed till birth of next child.

Uncontrolled hyperthyroidism, active thyroid eye disease especially in smokers, coexisting malignancy and non-compliance to radiation safety precautions are some other relative contraindications for therapy [47].

5.12 Side effects

Generally, RAI-131 therapy is well tolerated and majority of patients experience no side effects. However, some patients do experience adverse effect related to thyroid function, size, immunological response or as a result of extra-thyroidal irradiation.

Patients with large goiter may develop painful swelling of thyroid mimicking as sore throat lasting for up to 1 week following therapy. These symptoms are likely due to actinic thyroiditis i.e. result from radiation. It is usually managed with ice, NSAIDs and steroids if not resolved spontaneously. Slight discomfort of salivary (sialadenitis) with associated dry mouth (xerostomia) may occur in about 39% of the patients, but these are transient effects and permanent damage is very uncommon. Sialogogues or lemon juice can be used to accelerates radioiodine excretion by stimulating salivary glands resulting in approximately 40% reduction in dose to glands. This treatment should not be given in first 24 hours after therapy as it will result in increased absorbed dose due to rebound phenomena. Dry eyes (xerophthalmia) is very rare after radioiodine therapy. Mild leukopenia and thrombocytopenia can occur in some patients but it is usually temporary (6–10 weeks). Nausea and rarely vomiting can occurs immediately after therapy in some patients and resolve withing 24–72 hours [48].

Transient rise in serum thyroid hormones level may occur due to release of stored hormones leading to thyrotoxicosis. Cases of RAI-131 induced thyroid storm has also been reported with fatal outcome. This transient rise in hormone level depends on pre-treatment status. Patients who have been poorly controlled before therapy usually leads to exacerbation of hyperthyroidism requiring therapy. To reduce this risk, pre-treatment with ATD before therapy can be done to deplete intrathyroidal hormone stores [49].

Post-treatment hypothyroidism is an expected result following RAI-131 therapy indicating actual therapeutic response. Some authors consider it as a side effect of therapy. Recent ATA guidelines consider hypothyroidism the ultimate outcome of therapy and is more common in Grave's disease as compared to nodular thyroid disease. It may occur in early post-treatment period or develops gradually over a period of time. Delayed onset hypothyroidism incidence continues to increase with time after therapy at a rate of 4% per year in following year so that at 25 years nearly all patients become hypothyroid [41]. The ablative dosage concept for Grave's disease leads to thyroxin substitution in nearly all treated patients. In patients with toxic nodular thyroid disease incidence of hypothyroidism is greater in younger patients with age < 50 years in long-term follow-up. In general, majority of the patients usually follow transient hypothyroidism followed by euthyroidism and then permanent hypothyroidism after radioiodine therapy. Transient hypothyroidism is caused by disruption of normal hypothalamus-pituitary- thyroid axis and depletion of intra-thyroidal hormone stores.

Radioiodine induced thyroid damage can lead to immunological response due to release of thyroid autoantibodies peaking approximately 3–6 months after therapy. TRAb usually return to baseline within 1 year but remains detectable for many years. This thyroid autoimmunity results in thyroid associated orbitopathy, seen in approximately 15–30% of patients with Grave's disease and more common in patients with previous history of thyroid eye disease. The risk is associated with release of autoantibodies and development of hypothyroidism. Steroids have shown promising results in such cases. In patients with toxic or non-toxic nodular goiter, about 1–5% patients may develop de novo TRAb and occasionally orbitopathy. The risk is more pronounced in patients with previously circulating autoantibodies (TPO) and usually resolve spontaneously [48].

Fertility issues with radioiodine therapy are rare and late side effects. Some men may experience transient increase in gonadotropins and decrease spermatogenesis due to damage to germinal epithelium except in those receiving higher therapeutic doses in the range 200–300 mCi in whom permanent infertility may occur. Radiation dose associated with single ablative therapy does not cause permanent germinal epithelium damage, however patients requiring multiple therapy administration infertility can result due to cumulative dose effect. In such cases sperm storage can be considered. In female, about 20–30% experience menstrual abnormalities like amenorrhea or metrorrhagia lasting for 1 year and early menopause. RAI-131 therapy can also damage ovarian reserves in women treated at later ages [50].

Radioactive iodine therapy is thought to be associated with risk of developing cancer. This association has been extensively investigated and no convincing evidence could be established in development of thyroid cancer or secondary malignancies after therapy. A small negligible increase in relative risk of thyroid cancer after radioiodine therapy has been reported in some epidemiological studies. However, this seems to be associated with underlying thyroid disease rather the therapy itself. Some studies have reported the risk of developing secondary malignancies including stomach, kidney and breast after therapy and this risk is higher in patient with toxic nodular goiter. But this risk may be attributed to other confounding factors like age, smoking etc. Nevertheless, the risk of developing malignancy after therapy is negligible and needs further log-term studies [48, 51].

In patients with large goiter and retrosternal extension, tracheal compression can occur after therapy. In such cases therapy should be done in collaboration with otolaryngology department to address compressive emergency. Laryngeal edema, dysgeusia and recurrent laryngeal nerve palsy can occur rarely.

5.13 Radiation safety procedures

The amount of radiation received by a person from treated patient depends on activity retained in patient, distance and duration of contact. Mostly radioiodine therapy is administered as outpatient in registered and authorized facility. In case of indoor therapy, patient is released when no person is likely to receive greater than 5 mSv, when survey meter reading is less than 0.07 mSv/hour at 1 meter and when administered activity is less than 33 mCi or less. Before releasing the patient or after outdoor therapy, nuclear physician must instruct the patient on how to minimize unnecessary radiation exposure to surrounding people. Written information should also be provided.

Patient should be encouraged to drink plenty of water during first 8 hours and empty bladder frequently to eliminate excessive activity. Flush toilet twice and rinse sink and tub after use. Wash hands for 20 seconds. Maintain a distance of at least 3 feet from surrounding people for first 8 hours and use private car to drive home, if not possible maintain a distance of at least 3 feet from driver and passengers. Public transport should be avoided.

Do not share utensils, towels or wash clothes for 48 hours. Wash bed linen, towels and garments stained with urine, sweat or other body fluid. After washing these can be used by others.

Patient should sleep alone in separate room and avoid close physical contact for at least 7 days. Maintain a distance of 3–6 feet from pregnant females and children below 18 years of age. Infant and small children requiring nursing care should be provided with caretaker for at least 1 week. Avoid activities requiring close contact for more than 5 min for first week like public transport, movie theater, class room etc.

Both men and women should avoid pregnancy for at least 6 months. Breast feeding should not be resumed for current child. Small amount of radiation can trigger radiation sensors at airports, hospitals and sensitive buildings for up to 3 months. In such cases documentary proof regarding therapy can be obtained from concerned doctor [52].

6. Conclusion

Radioiodine therapy for hyperthyroidism is safe, cost-effective and efficient treatment modality. Patient selection, preparation and appropriate dose calculation to achieve desired therapeutic response are the corner stone of treatment. Post-therapy hypothyroidism should be anticipated and early initiation of thyroxin is associated with less clinical manifestations and also prevent worsening of orbitopathy.

Author details

Fida Hussain[1*], Muhammad Adil[1] and Mehmood Hussain[2]

1 Nuclear Medical Center, Armed Forces Institute of Pathology, Rawalpindi, Pakistan

2 Pak Emirates Military Hospital, Rawalpindi, Pakistan

*Address all correspondence to: fhsnmc@gmail.com

References

[1] Caputo M, Pecere A, Sarro A, Mele C, Ucciero A, Pagano L, et al. Incidence and prevalence of hyperthyroidism: A population-based study in the Piedmont region, Italy. Endocrine. 2020;**69**(1):107-112

[2] Taylor PN, Albrecht D, Scholz A, Gutierrez-Buey G, Lazarus JH, Dayan CM, et al. Global epidemiology of hyperthyroidism and hypothyroidism. Nature Reviews. Endocrinology. 2018;**14**:301-316

[3] Sánchez-Rodríguez MA, Castrejón-Delgado L, Zacarías-Flores M, Arronte-Rosales A, Mendoza-Núñez VM. Quality of life among post-menopausal women due to oxidative stress boosted by dysthymia and anxiety. BMC Women's Health. 2017;**17**(1):1-9

[4] Fahey FH, Grant FD, Thrall JH. Saul hertz, MD, and the birth of radionuclide therapy. EJNMMI Physics. 2017;**4**(1):1-7

[5] Okosieme OE, Taylor PN, Dayan CM. Should radioiodine now be first line treatment for graves' disease? Thyroid Research. 2020;**13**(1):1-7

[6] Rousset B, Dupuy C, Miot F, Dumont J. Thyroid Hormone Synthesis and Secretion. www.thyroidmanager.org. . Published by ENDOCRINE EDUCATION Inc, MA South Dartmouth, 2022 02748

[7] Sugimoto K, Mori K. Thyroid-Stimulating Hormone Regulation and Transcription in Hypothyroidism. In: Springer D, editor. Hypothyroidism - Influences and Treatments [Internet]. London: IntechOpen; 2012 [cited 2022 Oct 03] Available from: https://www.intechopen.com/chapters/27836 doi: 10.5772/32002

[8] Klein JR. The immune system as a regulator of thyroid hormone activity. Experimental Biology and Medicine. 2006;**231**(3):229-236

[9] Aghini-Lombardi F, Antonangeli L, Martino E, Vitti P, Maccherini D, Leoli F, et al. The spectrum of thyroid disorders in an iodine-deficient community: The Pescopagano survey. The Journal of Clinical Endocrinology & Metabolism. 1999;**84**(2):561-566

[10] Raheem N, Ahmed SA, Samaila MO. Histopathological pattern of thyroid diseases in Zaria: A 10-year review. Nigerian Postgraduate Medical Journal. 1 Jan 2018;**25**(1):37

[11] Sajjadi-Jazi SM, Sharifi F, Varmaghani M, Meybodi HA, Farzadfar F, Larijani B. Epidemiology of hyperthyroidism in Iran: A systematic review and meta-analysis. Journal of Diabetes & Metabolic Disorders. 2018;**17**(2):345-355

[12] Devereaux D, Tewelde SZ. Hyperthyroidism and thyrotoxicosis. Emergency Medicine Clinics. 2014;**32**(2):277-292

[13] Galindo RJ, Hurtado CR, Pasquel FJ, García Tome R, Peng L, Umpierrez GE. National trends in incidence, mortality, and clinical outcomes of patients hospitalized for thyrotoxicosis with and without thyroid storm in the United States, 2004-2013. Thyroid. 2019;**29**(1):36-43

[14] Antonelli A, Ferrari SM, Ragusa F, Elia G, Paparo SR, Ruffilli I, et al. Graves' disease: Epidemiology, genetic and environmental risk factors and viruses. Best Practice & Research Clinical Endocrinology & Metabolism. 2020;**34**(1):101387

[15] Khalid N, Can AS. Plummer disease. In: StatPearls [Internet]. Treasure Island (FL): StatPearls Publishing; 2022. Available from: https://www.ncbi.nlm.nih.gov/books/NBK565856/

[16] Mulita F, Anjum F. Thyroid Adenoma. In: StatPearls [Internet]. Treasure Island (FL): StatPearls Publishing; 2022. Available from: https://www.ncbi.nlm.nih.gov/books/NBK562252/

[17] Alfadda A, Sallam R, Elawad G, AlDhukair H, Alyahya M. Subacute thyroiditis: Clinical presentation and long term outcome. International Journal of Endocrinology. 2014;**2014**:1-7

[18] Hennessey JV. Subacute thyroiditis. In: Feingold KR, Anawalt B, Boyce A, et al., editors. Endotext [Internet]. South Dartmouth (MA): MDText.com, Inc.; 2000. Available from: https://www.ncbi.nlm.nih.gov/books/NBK279084/

[19] Samuels MH. Subacute, silent, and postpartum thyroiditis. The Medical Clinics of North America. 2012;**96**(2):223-233

[20] Sengul I, Sengul D, Pelikan A. Iodine induced hyperthyroidism: Do you mind? Sanamed. 2020;**15**(2):215-217

[21] Hammamy R, Farooqui K, Shariff M. Factitial hyperthyroidism: A diagnostic challenge. Authorea Preprints. 2021

[22] Bahn R, Burch H, Cooper D, Garber J, Greenlee M, Klein I, et al. Hyperthyroidism and other causes of thyrotoxicosis: Management guidelines of the American Thyroid Association and American Association of Clinical Endocrinologists. Thyroid. 2011;**21**(6):593-646

[23] Kahaly G, Bartalena L, Hegedüs L, Leenhardt L, Poppe K, Pearce S. 2018 European thyroid association guideline for the Management of Graves' hyperthyroidism. European Thyroid Journal. 2018;7(4):167-186

[24] Asban A, Dream S, Lindeman B. Is hyperthyroidism diagnosed and treated appropriately in the United States? Advances in Surgery. 2019;**53**:117-129

[25] McCready VR. Radioiodine—The success story of nuclear medicine. European Journal of Nuclear Medicine and Molecular Imaging. 2017;**44**:179-182

[26] Borges de Souza P, McCabe C. Radioiodine treatment: An historical and future perspective. Endocrine-Related Cancer. 2021;**28**(10):T121-T124

[27] Amdur RJ, Mazzaferri EL. Half-life and emission products of I-131. Essentials of Thyroid Cancer Management. Boston, MA: Springer; 2005 pp. 165-168

[28] Muhammad W. Radioactive iodine therapy for hyperthyroidism: Physics, treatment protocols and radiation protection. In: Handbook of Hyperthyroidism: Etiology, Diagnosis and Treatment. New York: Nova Science Publishers, Inc.; 2009. pp. 295-314

[29] Marzo K. Radiopharmaceuticals for Therapy of Thyroid Diseases. In: Bombardieri E, Seregni E, Evangelista L, Chiesa C, Chiti A, editors. Clinical Applications of Nuclear Medicine Targeted Therapy. Cham: Springer; 2018. Available from: https://doi.org/10.1007/978-3-319-63067-0_2

[30] Bombardieri E, Seregni E, Evangelista L, Chiesa C, Chiti A. Clinical Applications of Nuclear Medicine Targeted Therapy. 1st ed. Switzerland: Springer International Publishing; 2018

[31] Riley A, McKenzie G, Green V, Schettino G, England R, Greenman J. The effect of radioiodine treatment on

the diseased thyroid gland. International Journal of Radiation Biology. 2019;**95**(12):1718-1727

[32] Padda IS, Nguyen M. Radioactive iodine therapy. In: StatPearls [Internet]. Treasure Island (FL): StatPearls Publishing; 2022. Available from: https://www.ncbi.nlm.nih.gov/books/NBK557741/

[33] Nair D, Maweni R, Constantinou C, Kandiah S, Nagala S, Aung T. Clinical efficacy of fixed-dose radioactive iodine for the treatment of hyperthyroidism at a single Centre: Our experience. Irish Journal of Medical Science (1971). 2021;**191**(4):1659-1665

[34] Allahabadia A, Daykin J, Sheppard MC, Gough SC, Franklyn JA. Radioiodine treatment of hyperthyroidism prognostic factors for outcome. Journal of Clinical Endocrinology & Metabolism. 2001;**86**(8):3611-3617

[35] Pardo FJ, Serrano RL, Cases FJ, Peña MC, Crespo-Jara A, Vicente AM, et al. A prospective comparative study of two methods for the individual calculation of 131I activity in the treatment of hyperthyroidism. Endocrinología, Diabetes y Nutrición (English ed.). 2020;**67**(9):568-577

[36] Liu M, Jing D, Hu J, Yin S. Predictive factors of outcomes in personalized radioactive iodine (131I) treatment for graves' disease. The American Journal of the Medical Sciences. 2014;**348**(4):288-293

[37] Szumowski P, Mojsak M, Abdelrazek S, Sykała M, Amelian-Fiłonowicz A, Jurgilewicz D, et al. Calculation of therapeutic activity of radioiodine in graves' disease by means of Marinelli's formula, using technetium (99mTc) scintigraphy. Endocrine. 2016;**54**(3):751-756

[38] Dietlein M. Radioiodine therapy for benign thyroid disease. In: Clinical Nuclear Medicine. Cham: Springer; 2020. pp. 815-829

[39] Stagnaro-Green A, Abalovich M, Alexander E, Azizi F, Mestman J, Negro R, et al. Guidelines of the American Thyroid Association for the diagnosis and Management of Thyroid Disease during Pregnancy and Postpartum. Thyroid. 2011;**21**(10):1081-1125

[40] Laplano NE, Mercado-Asis LB. Recombinant TSH and lithium overcomes amiodarone-induced low radioiodine uptake in a thyrotoxic female. International Journal of Endocrinology and Metabolism. 2012;**10**(4):625

[41] Clarke SE. Radioiodine therapy for benign thyroid disease. In: Clinical Nuclear Medicine. Berlin, Heidelberg: Springer; 2007. pp. 409-417

[42] Silberstein E, Alavi A, Balon H, Clarke S, Divgi C, Gelfand M, et al. The SNMMI practice guideline for therapy of thyroid disease with 131I 3.0. Journal of Nuclear Medicine. 2012;**53**(10):1633-1651

[43] Aktolun C, Urhan M. Radioiodine therapy of benign thyroid diseases: Graves' disease, Plummer's disease, non-toxic goiter and nodules. In: Nuclear Medicine Therapy. New York, NY: Springer; 2013. pp. 281-314

[44] Kaplowitz PB, Jiang J, Vaidyanathan P. Radioactive iodine therapy for pediatric Graves' disease: A single-center experience over a 10-year period. Journal of Pediatric Endocrinology & Metabolism. 2020;**33**(3):383-389

[45] Hegedus L, Bonnema SJ, Bennedbaek FN. Management of simple nodular goiter: Current status and future perspectives. Endocrine Reviews. 2003;**24**(1):102-132

[46] Szumowski P, Abdelrazek S, Sykała M, Mojsak M, Żukowski Ł, Siewko K, et al. Enhancing the efficacy of 131I therapy in non-toxic multinodular goitre with appropriate use of methimazole: An analysis of randomized controlled study. Endocrine. 2020;**67**(1):136-142

[47] Gurgul E, Sowinski J. Primary hyperthyroidism—Diagnosis and treatment. Indications and contraindications for radioiodine therapy. Nuclear Medicine Review. 2011;**14**(1):29-32

[48] Bonnema SJ, Hegedüs L. Radioiodine therapy in benign thyroid diseases: Effects, side effects, and factors affecting therapeutic outcome. Endocrine Reviews. 2012;**33**(6):920-980

[49] McDermott MT, Kidd GS, Dodson LE Jr, Hofeldt FD. Radioiodine-induced thyroid storm: Case report and literature review. The American Journal of Medicine. 1983;**75**(2):353-359

[50] Navarro P, Rocher S, Miró-Martínez P, Oltra-Crespo S. Radioactive iodine and female fertility. Scientific Reports. 2022;**12**(1):1-7

[51] Lutterman S, Zwaveling-Soonawala N, Verberne H, Verburg F, van Trotsenburg A, Mooij C. The Efficacy and Short- and Long-Term Side Effects of Radioactive Iodine Treatment in Pediatric Graves' Disease: A Systematic Review. European Thyroid Journal. 2021;**10**(5):353-363

[52] Sisson TA, Freitas J, McDougall IR, Dauer LT, Hurley JR, Brierley JD, et al. Radiation safety in the treatment of patients with thyroid diseases by radioiodine 131I: Practice recommendations of the American Thyroid Association. Thyroid. 2011;**21**(4):335-346

Chapter 4

Therapeutic Options in Graves' Hyperthyroidism

Javaid Ahmad Bhat, Shoiab Mohd Patto, Pooran Sharma, Mohammad Hayat Bhat and Shahnaz Ahmad Mir

Abstract

The classical approach to treating Graves' hyperthyroidism involves rapid control of the symptoms, generally with a beta adrenergic blocker, and reduction of thyroid hormone secretion by antithyroid drugs (ATDs) and/or using one of the several modalities available, including radioactive iodine therapy (RAI), and surgery; the selection of the treatment modalities often varies according to different guidelines, patient preferences and local traditions. Thionamides are invariably used as first-line medication to control hyperthyroidism and induce remission of the disease, thereby relieving the symptoms. In case of failure of the medical therapy, which is not uncommon, definitive treatment with surgery or RAI is the standard modality of management after due consideration and discussion with the patients. However, the therapeutic options available for patients with Graves' hyperthyroidism have remained largely unchanged for the past several decades despite the current treatments having either limited efficacy or significant adverse effects. The clinical demand for new therapeutic regimens of Graves' disease has led to the emergence of several new therapeutic ideas/options like biologic, peptide immunomodulation and small molecules, currently under investigations which may lead to the restoration of a euthyroid state without the requirement for ongoing therapy, but the potential risk of immunocompromise and cost implications needs careful consideration.

Keywords: Graves' disease, anti-thyroid drugs, radioactive iodine, relapse and remission, thyroidectomy

1. Introduction

Graves' disease (GD) is an autoimmune thyroid disorders characterized by multi-systemic involvement, resulting from a complex interactions between genetic and environmental factors [1, 2]. It has an annual incidence of 20 to 50 cases per 100,000 individuals and is the most common cause of hyperthyroidism, accounting for 60–80% of the cases [3]. As with the other autoimmune diseases, women are affected more than men, with a peak incidence occurring between the age of 30 and 50 years, although no age is immune to the disease. It is estimated that approximately 0.5% of men and 3% of women develop Graves' disease during their lifetime [4]. Hyperthyroidism, diffuse goiter, and/or orbitopathy are the characteristic features of

GD, although involvement of other organ systems is not rare. The age of the patient, severity and duration of the disease, determine the presentation and the course of the disease [5]. variety of characteristic symptoms and physical findings of the disease either results from hyperthyroidism (goiter in certain cases) or is a consequence of underlying autoimmunity [6]. Impaired quality of life, work disability [7, 8] and an increased risk of death [9] associated with GD render it imperative to understand the effectiveness of the different modalities of treatment available for the GD to acheive lasting euthyroidism for a favorable outcome. Clinical and biochemical features associated with elevated levels of thyroid hormone, particularly of a long duration and/or orbitopathy, elevated levels of TSH-receptor antibodies (TRAbs) along with a diffuse increase in radioactive iodine or technetium uptake scan, confirm the diagnosis of GD. The association of GD with plethora of systemic manifestations, including typical and atypical, and a relatively prolonged course on account of higher rates of recurrences and relapse responsible for significant morbidity and an increased risk of mortality warrant proper management of the disease and the associated complications [10]. The treatment for GD comprises rapid control of the symptoms, generally with a beta adrenergic blocker, and reduction of thyroid hormone levels using one of the several modalities available, including ATDs to block thyroid hormone synthesis, destruction of the thyroid gland by RAI, and or removal of thyroid gland by surgery respectively; the selection of the optimal approach often varies according to the patient preference, different guidelines, clinical factors and local traditions. The therapeutic options available for patients with Graves' hyperthyroidism have to some extent been successful in reliving the patients of signs and symptoms but lack of efficacy of ATDs in successful maintenance of remission after stopping these drugs in many patients and/or need for lifelong thyroid hormone replacement on account of the lack of functional thyroid tissue in patients treated with either radioiodine, or surgery and improvement in quality of life of in some patients has led to the need for newer therapeutic options with better disease outcome and improved degree of morbidity and mortality. The demand for new therapeutic options, combined with greater insight into basic immunobiology, has led to the emergence of novel approaches to treat Graves' disease. The novel therapeutic options under investigations like biologic, peptide immunomodulation and small molecule, may lead to the restoration of a euthyroid state without the requirement for ongoing therapy, but the potential risk of immunocompromise and cost implications needs careful consideration.

In this chapter we try to dwell upon the traditional treatment options, such as antithyroid drugs, radioiodine and or thyroidectomy, available for Graves' hyperthyroidism, besides new strategies under investigation and summarize the effective components of different modalities of management to restore euthyroidism for a favorable outcome of the disease.

2. Management options for Graves' disease

The management of GD has been largely directed towards controlling the hyperthyroidism despite the autoimmune mechanisms responsible for the syndrome. Treatment involves alleviation of symptoms and correction of the thyrotoxic state. Adrenergic hyperfunction is treated with beta-adrenergic blockade. Correcting the excessive thyroid hormone levels can be accomplished with antithyroid medications that block the synthesis of thyroid hormones or by treatment with radioactive iodine and surgery resulting in loss of functional thyroid tissue. The therapeutic options available are: (I) antithyroid drug therapy, (II) surgery, and (III) radioiodine. These modalities are safe and cost-effective and can be the first-line treatment for hyperthyroidism not only due to GD, but also due to toxic adenoma, and toxic multinodular goiter [11]. Despite the use of these three treatments for decades, selection of the optimal therapy for GD still poses a challenge for both the physician and the patient. Each modality has its unique advantages and disadvantages with no single best therapy for all patients. A prudent approach is to make a selection after a thoughtful discussion with the patient regarding advantages, risks, and cost-effectiveness, taking into consideration the values and preferences of the patient. Autoimmune nature of the disease and lack of treatment to address the underlying autoimmune pathogenesis has turned the research focus on the potential use of immunotherapy in GD [12]. Despite the good understanding of the underlying mechanism, it is worth mentioning that the selection of the right therapy for each patient still poses a challenge to the clinician as there is no single best therapy for all patients [13].

3. Antithyroid drugs therapy for GD

ATD are used as first line therapy in the majority of patients and represent the predominant therapy in Europe, Asia, and as bridge therapy in the USA [12]. The main ATDs are thionamides, such as carbimazole (CBZ), methimazole (MMI) the active metabolite of the CBZ and propylthiouracil (PTU). CBZ, a prodrug molecule needs decarboxylation in the liver to get converted to its active substance MMI. Thionamides block the formation of thyroid hormone T3 and T4 by inhibiting enzyme thyroid peroxidase. A 12- to 18-month course of antithyroid drugs may lead to a remission in approximately 50% of patients with theoretically significant (albeit rare) adverse reactions.

Thyroid gland plays the central role in the metabolism of iodine and synthesis of thyroid hormones such as T3 and T4. Thyroid follicular cells take up the iodine from blood stream through an active transport system constituted by a transporting protein sodium iodide symporter (NIS) which is located at the basolateral membrane of these follicular cells. This iodine is used for the process of iodination whereby iodine binds to tyrosine molecule of thyroglobulin (Tg) promoted by enzyme thyroid peroxidase. The process of iodination of tyrosine molecules leads to the formation of 3-monoiodotyrosine (MIT) and 3, 5-diiodotyrosine (DIT) which is coupled afterwards leading to the formation of thyroid hormones. Triiodothyronine (T3) hormone is formed by coupling of one molecule each of MIT and DIT and thyroxine (T4) hormone is formed by coupling of two DIT molecules. These thyroid hormones are stored in the thyroid cells as colloid in a quantity enough to meet the body requirements for up to 3 months. The whole process of formation of thyroid hormones is regulated by thyroid stimulating hormone (TSH) released from anterior pituitary gland which stimulates the expression of NIS through TSH receptor (TSH-R) which then activates follicular cells. The uptake and metabolism of the radioactive iodine (I-123 and I-131) follows the same process as nutritional iodine to get incorporated into the thyroid hormones [13].

Thionamide drugs are actively transported into the thyroid where they serve as the preferential substrate for the iodinating intermediate of thyroid peroxidase and thus interfere with the iodination of tyrosine resulting in inhibition of the synthesis of T3 and T_4 hormones. This whole process results in the diversion of oxidized iodine from the tyrosyl iodination sites in thyroglobulin. Thionamides also inhibit the coupling of iodothyronines and hence reduce the biosynthesis of thyroid hormones [14]. In addition, PTU also blocks extrathyroidal deiodination of T4 to T3 resulting in less conversion of T4 to T3, but this process of peripheral inhibition is of little clinical significance other than perhaps in the management of thyrotoxic crisis, when it is important to lower the raised serum T_3 concentration as quickly as possible.

ATDs are indicated as a first-line treatment of GD, particularly in younger subjects, and also for short-term treatment of GD before definitive therapy with RAI or thyroidectomy [6]. Available only as oral preparations, they however, have been used as retention enemas in patients in whom oral intake is not possible or is contraindicated. Alteration of intrathyroidal immunoregulatory mechanisms have been reported with ATDs which is believed to contribute to long term success of maintenance of disease remission. In addition they have been reported to have immunosuppressive effect resulting in reduction of TSHR-Ab levels, soluble IL-2 receptor (sIL-2R) and intercellular adhesion molecule-1 (ICAM-1) [15]. However, this immunomodulatory effect has proved to be short-lived as is evident from the presence of frequent relapse of Graves' hyperthyroidism in patients after drug withdrawal.

Historically, CBZ has been the drug of choice in the United Kingdom, but in all other areas of the world, MMI has been the drug of choice. The use of PTU is restricted to first trimester of pregnancy and in patients who have reacted adversely to CBZ or MMI and is also widely employed in the America.

ATDs are given consideration as first line therapy in the following category of patients with Graves' disease [16].

a. Younger patients

b. Bridge therapy as short term treatment prior to RAI or surgery.

c. Patients with mild disease (small size of goiter, negative or low TRAbs values),

d. Elderly comorbid patients at high risk of postoperative complications

e. Patients with a history of head and neck irradiation or surgery.

f. GD in pregnancy.

g. Rapid biochemical control in moderate to severe active Graves' orbitopathy (GO)

h. Lack of access to an experienced thyroid surgeon.

3.1 Carbimazole

Carbimazole, a pro-drug on oral administration is converted to methimazole in liver which is an active substance. Historically, CBZ has been the drug of choice in the United Kingdom and is also available in Europe, but is not approved for use in the United States. Conversion to active substance methimazole is rapid and almost complete either in the gastrointestinal tract or immediately on absorption, as is evident from the observation that only drug concentrations of methimazole but not carbimazole are detected in the serum and thyroid gland after ingestion. Ten milligrams of carbimazole is equivalent to 6 mg of methimazole. Carbimazole acts as the substrate for thyroid peroxidase (TPO) and decrease the incorporation of iodide into tyrosine molecules. In addition, it also inhibits coupling of iodinated precursor molecules like mono-iodinated and di-iodinated residues to form T_4 and T_3 hormones.

Carbimazole has been preferred in some patients on account of fewer side effects such as less frequent gastrointestinal problems compared with methimazole. The starting dose of CBZ is usually between 20 to 40 mg/day depending on the severity of the hyperthyroidism. The initial high dose of the drugs can be tapered down after 4 to 8 weeks in what is referred to as the titration regimen. A maintenance dose of 5 to 20 mg of CBZ is achieved by about 4 to 6 months and this is continued for 12 to 18 months. Once a patient is on a maintenance dose of CBZ, thyroid hormone assessment is done every 2 to 4 months and the treatment continued for 12 to 18 months depending on the response to achieve the immunomodulatory role of the drug to reduce the rate of recurrence of the disease. The patients are followed on regular basis based on thyroid hormone levels and clinical status of the patient. Some studies have also advocated block and replacement regimen to avoid severe hypothyroidism during treatment where CBZ/MMI in dose of 30–50 mg daily along with thyroxin replacement is used throughout the coarse but side effects of ATD are more with this kind of regimen [17].

3.1.1 Adverse effects

Adverse effects associated with the use of antithyroid medication range from milder adverse events such subcutaneous eruptions, gastrointestinal disorders and arthralgia's to more serious complications as agranulocytosis, frank polyarthritis and hepatotoxicity (Explained in Section 2.1.2).

3.2 Methimazole

Methimazole, an antithyroid drug is an active metabolite of carbimazole- a pro-drug, which belongs to the thionamide class. On entering the blood stream following oral administration, methimazole inhibits the enzyme thyroid peroxidase and thus decrease the incorporation of iodide into tyrosine residues of thyroglobulin resulting in the inhibition of the synthesis of thyroid hormones T4 and T3. Methimazole also inhibits oxidation of iodine and the coupling of iodotyrosyl residues and thus blocks the production of thyroid hormone [18].

The first line of therapeutic option for the treatment of Graves hyperthyroidism is usually Methimazole with few exceptions, due to the lower risk of hepatotoxicity compared to propylthiouracil [18]. Methimazole is usually the started from 10 to 30 mg daily in divided doses, with titration and variable maintenance doses depending on the severity of hyperthyroidism. As the disease goes in remission, dose is gradually reduced through the course of disease based on severity of the illness referred as "titration regimen". Thyroid function tests are done at 6–8 weekly intervals after initial treatment, and the dose is titrated based on T4 and T3 hormone levels. The levels of T3 & T4 are more reliable to guide the dosage of antithyroid drugs as the TSH values remain suppressed for long time. The oral route of administration and non-requirement dose adjustment except in patients with severe hepatic impairment makes the of MMI drug of choice worth consideration as ATD [18]. With the half-life exceeding 6 hours in follicular cells [19, 20], the administration of MMI in a single daily dose is considered to be effective [21, 22]. The patients with thyroid storm, require higher doses, with a starting dose of 60 to 80 mg per day with the dose divided every 4 to 8 hours, with a maximum dose of 120 mg [23].

Once a patient is on a maintenance dose of MMI, thyroid hormone assessment is done every 2 to 4 months and the treatment continued for 12 to 18 months depending on the response to achieve the immunomodulatory role of the drug to reduce the rate of recurrence of the disease.

3.2.1 Adverse effects

The adverse effects are usually not so common but serious drug reactions of methimazole seem to be dose related (40 mg/day or more). These adverse drug effects include agranulocytosis, hepatotoxicity, and teratogenicity [24].

Agranulocytosis can occur at any time during the course of MMI therapy but usually occurs in the first few months of initiation. Absolute granulocyte count of less than 500 per ml, fever and sore throat characterize the agranulocytosis. Patients are advised to stop the medication and report to the hospital for further management in case of development of such symptom. Treatment consists of stopping methimazole if the granulocyte count is less than 1000 per ml and give antibiotic treatment. Methimazole associated agranulocytosis predicts the risk of agranulocytosis due to propylthiouracil, thus necessitating the circumventing of the use of propylthiouracil in these patients.

Cholestasis characterize the MMI associated hepatotoxicity and is dose independent and shows slow recovery after discontinuation of the drug [25].

The teratogenic effects of MMI include aplasia cutis, facial dysmorphism, esophageal and choanal atresia, umbilical malformations as well as craniofacial malformations and are result of free placental crossing of the drug, especially in the first trimester. For this reason, the use of propylthiouracil in the first trimester of pregnancy is preferred [25, 26].

3.3 Propylthiouracil

Propylthiouracil is an antithyroid drug that is mostly used as a second treatment option in hyperthyroidism after MMI/CBZ owing to higher risk of hepatotoxicity. In patients with a contraindication to CBZ/MMI or radioactive iodine therapy, propylthiouracil provides an option to be used as second line treatment option. Propylthiouracil is however, preferred as the first line of treatment in patients with thyroid storm because of its greater efficacy on account of inhibition of the thyroid deiodinase resulting in the peripheral conversion of T4 to T3. Similarly in the first trimester of pregnancy, propylthiouracil is favored because of the relatively lower teratogenic profile compared to methimazole [25].

Propylthiouracil acts by inhibition of thyroid peroxidase, enzyme responsible for oxidization of iodine and its incorporation into the tyrosine molecule, resulting in inhibition of the formation of monoiodothyronine and diiodotyrosine. Unlike methimazole, propylthiouracil causes peripheral inhibition in conversion of T4 to T3 by inhibiting the enzyme deiodinase [25, 26].

The drug like CBZ is also available only as an oral preparation. The severity of the hyperthyroidism usually guides the starting dose of the propylthiouracil. The usual starting dose is 300 mg daily divided every 8 hours, with titration of the dose up to a maximum dose of 600 to 900 mg daily. However, the usual dose of propylthiouracil in patients with thyroid storm is 500 to 1000 mg daily divided every 4 hours [25, 26]. Once patient is euthyroid, the maintenance dose of propylthiouracil is around 100 to 150 mg per day.

3.3.1 Adverse effects

U.S. Food and Drug Administration's has issued a box warning highlighting higher risk of severe liver injury associated with use of propylthiouracil. As a consequence of this serious adverse effect, CBZ/MMI is preferred as first line of treatment except in patients with an adverse drug reaction to CBZ/MMI and during the first trimester of pregnancy [27, 28]. However, adverse effects of propylthiouracil has not been associated with the dose of drug unlike methimazole [24]. Hepatic injury and acute viral hepatitis like syndrome is one of the most perturbing adverse drug effects of the propylthiouracil, arising 2 to 12 weeks after starting the medication. These adverse drug reactions can occur at any time during the course of treatment but are usually observed during the first 6 months of treatment. The specific symptoms along with raised liver enzymes point to the initial diagnosis. The injury can be severe and many fatal cases have been described. The presence higher risk of hepatotoxicity in pregnancy, excludes the use of methimazole in the first trimester [25, 26].

ANCA-associated vasculitis has been associated with the use of propylthiouracil and is responsible for conditions like glomerulonephritis, alveolar hemorrhage, central nervous system compromise, and leukocytoclastic vasculitis. These conditions though less frequent, may be responsible for significant morbidity and may improve upon drug withdrawal or require additional immunosuppressive treatment [25, 26].

Agranulocytosis as an adverse reaction is seen in up to 0.5% of patients, especially in the first 3 months of treatment. The agranulocytosis may manifest with symptoms like sore throat, fever and decrease in absolute granulocyte count. Patient are educated about the possibility of this condition and instructed to stop the medication and report to the hospital for further management.

Hypersensitivity, interstitial nephritis, hypothyroidism, aplastic anemia and potential teratogenicity are the other adverse effects seen with use of propylthiouracil [25, 26].

4. Radioiodine therapy

Radioactive iodine has been used for several decades to treat thyroid disorders (both malignant and benign) and preferred first-line treatment in many cases like GD. A safe and effective management modality, RAI is used as definitive treatment for GD except for the development or worsening of thyroid eye disease in approximately 15–20% of patients [29]. RAI in GD involves systemic administration of I-131 for selective irradiation of hyper functioning thyroid gland. Radioiodine on administration is taken up by thyroid gland and is incorporated into the thyroid hormones. Ionizing damage and tissue necrosis by radioiodine is responsible for destruction of the follicle cells of the hyper functioning thyroid gland resulting in an eventual ablation of functional thyroid tissue and thus providing a definite therapy of hyperthyroidism thereby improving patient's quality of life.

Exacerbation of underlying orbitopathy apart, radioiodine therapy is well tolerated with fewer complications. The safety and efficacy of radioiodine treatment and the several beneficial effects over thyroid surgery and ATDs have been documented and are widely accepted. A beta-emitting radionuclide with a physical half-life of 8.4 days, I-131 is the radionuclide of choice to treat thyroid disorders. Beta-minus decay of I-131 results in emission of high-energy beta particles which are responsible for high radiation, particularly to the thyroid follicular cells, gradually leading to the destruction of these cells manifesting as volume reduction and therapy outcome in GD.

Radioiodine mediated radiobiological effects are the result of the DNA damage effected through breakage of molecular bonds, and/or through the formation of free radicals leading to genetic damage, mutations, or cell death. This leads to a decrease production of thyroid hormones and/or reduction in the size of thyroid gland. However, there are no ideal methods of predicting the clinical response or of measuring the individual radio sensitivity to RAI therapy [30].

RAI has been the most preferable treatment in USA for many years, but currently there is a tendency towards ATD therapy on account of being safe and definitive therapy for GD. The goal of RAI treatment is to radiate thyroid cells to render the patient euthyroid using low doses of I-131. Hypothyroidism being an inevitable and unpredictable progressive outcome of RAI treatment, is the desired result of RAI treatment and considered as the elimination of hyperthyroidism [31]. Though the RAI therapy is safe and effective and is considered as first line therapy in many cases but is preferably indicated for individuals who are at higher risk of surgical complications, or in those with a history of prior surgery or irradiation of the head and neck, previously operated, and after failure of ATD therapy to control hyperthyroidism and/or contraindications to ATD therapy. Similarly it is preferred modality of choice in the absence of access to an experienced thyroid surgeon and in patients with right heart failure, periodic thyrotoxic hypokalemic paralysis, congestive heart failure or pulmonary hypertension [16].

Radioablation is contraindicated in pregnant and breastfeeding women, inability to follow radiation safety rules, suspicion of thyroid cancer and in moderate to severe orbitopathy [16]. Female patients of childbearing age should undergo a pregnancy test 3 days prior to radioiodine administration and provide written signed declaration confirming the non-pregnant status. Serum pregnancy test being more sensitive is preferable to urine test [32].

Patients should be advised against the conception 6 months post RAI therapy. RAI therapy should be administrated 6 weeks to 3 months after lactation is disrupted [33].

Patients must be instructed to discontinue use of all iodine containing medications and be placed on an iodine-restricted diet in order to increase radioiodine uptake (RAIU) and thus to have desired therapeutic effect. Withdrawal of ATD for 3–7 days and iodine restriction for 1 to 2 weeks before RAI administration is also recommended.

RAI administration in hyperthyroidism provides symptomatic relief within weeks. To avoid increased failure rate and reduced the rates of hypothyroidism, ATDs can be withheld for 3–7 days before and after radioiodine administration [15, 34]. Patients at a higher risk of cardiac complications especially rhythm disturbances due to severe hyperthyroidism should be put on B-adrenergic blockade.

RAI treatment may experience some side effects of radioiodine therapy despite being considered safe. Post radiation thyroiditis an adverse effect of radiation treatment manifest as transient elevation of thyroid hormones resulting in exacerbation of hyperthyroid symptoms. The risk of eventual hypothyroidism though a desired result, is high especially after treatment of GD. However, the most undesirable and potentially troublesome adverse radiation effect is potential worsening of thyroid associated ophthalmopathy. Therefore, a close monitoring of the thyroid function is warranted to detect hypothyroidism earlier on in order to be treated as soon as possible.

Post radioiodine therapy thyroid hormones return to normal levels in the majority of the patients while resolution of clinical symptoms is observed in 4–8 weeks post therapy. Hypothyroidism sets in more than 80% of the patients 16 weeks post RAI therapy. The post radiation hypothyroidism is usually permanent however, in rare cases it may be transient and the patient may return to a euthyroid state or remain hyperthyroid. In the latter scenario there is no decrease of patients thyroid size [16]. Factors observed to affect the outcome of RAI treatment include thyroid size, iodine intake (diet or iodine containing medicine), dose regimens, compensation of hyperthyroidism, and the timing of the withdrawal of ATDs.

To assess the efficacy of the radioiodine treatment and timely detection of developing hypothyroidism or persistent hyperthyroidism close monitoring of the thyroid function is essential for favorable outcome. The review of thyroid function should be carried out within 1–2 months by assessing the values of serum TSH, FT4 and FT3 to be repeated every 4–6 weeks for the first 6 months or until the patient becomes hypothyroid and is stable on levothyroxine replacement [35].

5. Surgery

Thyroidectomy is the oldest and the preferred modality of treatment for Graves' disease and has been found to be at par with ATDs and radioiodine in reducing the serum thyroid hormone levels with normalization of hormone levels within 6 weeks of therapy [36]. The role of thyroid surgery particularly as an alternative to ATD in uncontrolled hyperthyroidism despite being on higher drug doses or in cases of recurrent hyperthyroidism is an attractive option. Surgical management again is a preferred option for patients in few conditions, such as in patients with large goiters with compressive symptoms, women desirous of conception shortly after treatment, younger patients with high risk of recurrence following medical management, nodular thyroid where malignancy may coexist. Patient's undergone surgical thyroidectomy is advised against the conception till they achieve euthyroidism either spontaneously or with levothyroxine replacement therapy. The surgical thyroidectomy does not appear to affect the course of Graves ophthalmopathy thus risk of its exacerbation and as such preferred mode of management in severe Graves' ophthalmopathy. Failure of antithyroid medications or radio-iodine therapy and patient preference to surgical approach are the other indication for thyroid surgery so are the patients who do not want the exposure to antithyroid drugs or radioiodine.

5.1 Preoperative management

The patients must reach euthyroidism to achieve hemodynamic stability, before they can undergo surgery. This will reduce the risk of complications [6, 37]. Preparation for surgery involves use of [38]:

1. Beta blockers such as propranolol (40–120 mg/day) or atenolol (25–50 mg/day) should be used until patient is clinically euthyroid that is thyroid function levels are within the normal limits

2. ATD therapy is used up until the day of surgery.

3. Use of potassium iodide (KI), saturated solution of potassium iodide (SSKI), or Lugol solution preoperatively have been shown to decrease the vascularity of the gland, thyroid blood flow and intraoperative blood loss beside acute inhibitory

effects of iodide on new thyroid hormone synthesis, referred to as the Wolff-Chaikoff effect. However, use of iodide products has not been associated with change in outcomes in few studies.

3.1 SSKI is used as 1 to 2 drops (50 mg/drop) TID and should be initiated 7 to 10 days prior to surgery and discontinued on the day of surgery.

3.2 Similarly Lugol solution (KI-iodine solution) as 5 to 7 drops (8 mg iodide/iodine per drop) daily can also be used as alternative [16].

3.3 In addition, corticosteroid like betamethasone 0.5 mg every 6 hours) or dexamethasone (2 mg orally or intravenously 4 times daily) and cholestyramine (4 grams six hourly) can be used for rapid preparation for emergent surgery to avoid the risk of thyroid storm.

Although preoperative use of these compounds has been advocated by ATA guidelines, the advantages of use of these agents preoperatively on the outcome of surgery is still debated.

4. The pre-op levels of serum calcium and vitamin D levels should be determined to establish a baseline level. Replacement therapy should be instituted if low to avoid post op hypocalcemia.

5. Postoperatively serum calcium, albumin and parathyroid hormone levels should be measured to screen for postop hypocalcemia so to have earlier detection of transient and later permanent hypoparathyroidism

6. Pre-op substitution of calcium carbonate in the dosages of 1gram for 3 weeks prior the procedure can avoid postoperative hypocalcemia.

7. Postoperatively all patients should be advised to have 1gram calcium carbonate three times a day for 2 weeks until the normalization of calcium and parathyroid hormone (PTH) levels are documented.

5.2 Total thyroidectomy versus subtotal thyroidectomy

Total thyroidectomy (removal all of the thyroid tissue) is preferred to subtotal thyroidectomy (leaving 4 to 7 grams of thyroid). The extent of thyroid resection in GD remains controversial. Total thyroidectomy versus subtotal thyroidectomy is a balance between risk of recurrence of hyperthyroidism in case of subtotal thyroidectomy and incidence of hypothyroidism seen with total thyroidectomy [38]. Total thyroidectomy is given the preference to subtotal thyroidectomy to avoid the risk of recurrence at the cost of rendering the patient on the side of hypothyroidism, in addition to avoid the second surgery to remove the residual tissue, which will be more difficult on account of scar tissue formation and distortion of tissue planes with prior surgery i.e., subtotal thyroidectomy [39]. In a systematic review and meta-analysis of total vs. subtotal thyroidectomy for GD by Feroci et al., the odds ratio (OR) of transient and permanent hypoparathyroidism favors subtotal thyroidectomy, the OR of the recurrence of hyperthyroidism favors total thyroidectomy [37]. One of the randomized trials involving 191 patients of GD by Barczynski et al., compared total thyroidectomy vs. subtotal thyroidectomy and followed these patients over a span of 5 years. Patients undergoing total thyroidectomy had a complete remission of the disease and lower risk of hypoparathyroidism (transient and or permanent) compared to subtotal thyroidectomy cohort [39].

Total thyroidectomy offers a better chance of cure of hyperthyroidism than bilateral subtotal thyroidectomy despite the controversy regarding the extent of thyroid resection in GD and can be accomplished safely with slight increase in the risk of temporary and permanent hypoparathyroidism.

Total thyroidectomy has been endorsed as the procedure of choice for the surgical management of GD [40] despite other studies [41, 42] arguing that subtotal thyroidectomy especially when performed with a remnant thyroid tissue of less than 3 gm, may allow permanent cure of hyperthyroidism to ensure euthyroid state in a significant proportion of patients with lower risk of recurrent hyperthyroidism [43].

5.2.1 Complications

Nonfatal complications associated with surgery are hypoparathyroidism either permanent (1–3%) or transient (10%) and vocal cord paralysis and hypothyroidism.

6. Management of Graves' disease during pregnancy

Graves' disease affects approximately 0.1% of pregnancies and if inadequately treated carries a substantial risk of adverse effects in both mother and child [44]. Untreated hyperthyroidism results in increased risk of pre-eclampsia, preterm delivery, low birth weight and increased neonatal mortality and morbidity. The mother is also at increased risk of heart failure, thyroid storm and pre-eclampsia. Changes in thyroid hormone concentrations that are characteristic of hyperthyroidism must be distinguished from gestational thyrotoxicosis affecting as many as 20% of pregnancies resulting TSH receptor stimulation by elevated serum levels of human chorionic gonadotropin (hCG), especially in the first trimester to ensure the early recognition and management to have a favorable outcome. Fetal hyperthyroidism can be life-threatening, and needs to be recognized as soon as possible so that treatment of the fetus with antithyroid drugs via the mother can be initiated. Antithyroid drug treatment of hyperthyroidism in pregnant women is controversial because in utero exposure with the usual ATDs especially methimazole and/or carbimazole have been the associated with between severe birth defects and the alternative propylthiouracil with hepatotoxicity. As both propylthiouracil and methimazole are associated with birth defects, lowest effective dose of an antithyroid drug should be used to maintain thyroid function at the upper limit of the normal range in order to avoid overtreatment and subsequent fetal hypothyroidism [45]. The use of propylthiouracil in the first trimester and methimazole during the remainder of pregnancy is currently recommended on the basis of a consideration of potentially severe birth defects.

Thyroid function should be monitored monthly. In up to 50% of cases, antithyroid drugs may be discontinued after the first trimester as GD improves spontaneously during pregnancy, but postpartum relapse is common due to a rebound in autoimmunity [44]. Elevated Thyrotropin-receptor antibodies levels especially by a factor of more than 3 in the third trimester, identifies pregnancies at risk for neonatal hyperthyroidism [44]. Breast-feeding is safe with either methimazole or propylthiouracil, but methimazole is recommended for postpartum therapy and does not affect infant thyroid function in the doses commonly used [46, 47].

PTU is the preferred antithyroid agent during pregnancy, as congenital anomalies such as aplasia cutis (single or multiple lesions of 0.5 to 3 cm at the vertex or occipital area in the scalp), choanal and esophageal atresia are reported more frequently with MMI [48]. However, the incidence of these anomalies is quite rare and it is acceptable to continue MMI particularly in areas where PTU is not easily available. The PTU dosage is reduced to the lowest effective dose to maintain the fT4 towards the upper end of the reference range with monthly monitoring of thyroid functions [49]. The activity levels of Graves' disease may fluctuate during pregnancy, with exacerbation during the first trimester with improvement in later pregnancy with a higher chance of an exacerbation soon after delivery. Therefore, thyroid function should be monitored every 2 to 3 months for 1 year following delivery to detect early relapse.

7. Newer therapeutic options

Newer treatment options based on antigen-specific Immunotherapy, immunobiology such as biologics, small molecules and peptide immunomodulation under investigations are in different stages of development particularly aimed at achieving euthyroidism without the requirement for ongoing therapy.

7.1 Antigen-specific immunotherapy

The antigen-specific immunotherapies are intended to restore the immune tolerance to the immunodominant epitopes responsible for the aberrant autoimmune response. Lack of generalized immunosuppression and skewing of the immune response associated with these therapies pose no greater risk of infection or different immune-mediated conditions. A study by Pearce et al., investigated a combination of two TSHR peptides (ATX-GD-59) in 12 subjects with mild-to-moderate untreated hyperthyroidism that was administered 10 times to each participant over 18 weeks by intradermal injection, in 12 subjects with mild-to-moderate untreated hyperthyroidism. The treatment was also well tolerated, with 10/12 participants finishing the study and 7/10 subjects had improvement in their thyroid function over the 18 weeks of ATX-GD-59, with 50% normalizing their serum fT3 concentrations, reduction in serum TSHR autoantibodies suggesting that ATX-GD-59 may have a significant potential for effective disease-modifying therapeutic cure in GD [50].

7.2 Immunomodulation

Immunomodulation of B lymphocytes by directly targeting the B cells or their associated interactors and cytokines by molecules such as iscalimab (anti-CD40), belimumab (anti-BAFF), and rituximab (anti-CD20).

7.3 Blocking of signaling

Blocking of signaling of TSH receptors by small molecular TSHR antagonist and *TSHR stimulation by TSH or TRAbs* (K1–70 blocking),

7.4 Inhibition of immunoglobulin

Inhibition of immunoglobulin recycling by blocking the neonatal Fc receptor (efgartigimod and rozanolixizumab), which recycles endocytosed IgG antibody by binding it in the acidic conditions of the lysosome and recycling it to the cell membrane for release back into the circulation [51].

These newer therapies may dawn the era of restoring a euthyroid state in the patients of GD without the need for ongoing therapy with least potential risks such as immunocompromise and render destructive radioiodine thyroid ablation and thyroidectomy obsolete.

8. Conclusions

The treatment of Graves' disease, a most common cause of hyperthyroidism should be tailored to the specific needs of each patient with the benefits and risks of each therapy explained in full. Antithyroid drugs, surgery and radioactive iodine are still therapeutic options of choice and are widely available and exercised. Antithyroid drugs continue to be the first line of treatment, except for patients with contraindications or intolerance. Surgical ablation is still an option in a smaller proportion of patients with particular conditions. Radioactive iodine therapy has gained more acceptability and in many cases it is preferred first-line treatment. RAI is a safe and effective definitive treatment for GD.

New treatment options with biological and immunomodulatory therapy are under development and in the future may be a treatment option with a lower risk of toxicity and perhaps higher rates of cure.

Conflict of interest

There is no conflict of interest.

Author details

Javaid Ahmad Bhat*, Shoiab Mohd Patto, Pooran Sharma, Mohammad Hayat Bhat and Shahnaz Ahmad Mir
Department of Endocrinology, Superspeciality Hospital, Shireen Bagh, Srinagar, Kashmir, India

*Address all correspondence to: javaidrasool@rediffmail.com

References

[1] Tomer Y. Mechanisms of autoimmune thyroid diseases: From genetics to epigenetics. Annual Review of Pathology. 2014;**9**:147-156

[2] Brix TH, Kyvik KO, Christensen K, Hegedüs L. Evidence for a major role of heredity in Graves' disease: A population-based study of two Danish twin cohorts. The Journal of Clinical Endocrinology and Metabolism. 2001;**86**(2):930-934

[3] Zimmermann MB, Boelaert K. Iodine deficiency and thyroid disorders. The Lancet Diabetes and Endocrinology. 2015;**3**(4):286-295

[4] Nyström HF, Jansson S, Berg G. Incidence rate and clinical features of hyperthyroidism in a long-term iodine sufficient area of Sweden (Gothenburg) 2003-2005. Clinical Endocrinology. 2013;**78**(5):768-776

[5] Nordyke RA, Gilbert FI, Harada AS. Graves' disease. Influence of age on clinical findings. Archives of Internal Medicine. 1988;**148**(3):626-631

[6] Smith TJ, Hegedüs L. Graves' Disease. The New England Journal of Medicine. 2016;**375**(16):1552-1565

[7] Kahaly GJ, Petrak F, Hardt J, Pitz S, Egle UT. Psychosocial morbidity of Graves' orbitopathy. Clinical Endocrinology. 2005;**63**(4):395-402

[8] Brandt F, Thvilum M, Hegedüs L, Brix TH. Hyperthyroidism is associated with work disability and loss of labour market income. A Danish register-based study in singletons and disease-discordant twin pairs. European Journal of Endocrinology. 2015;**173**(5):595-602

[9] Brandt F, Almind D, Christensen K, Green A, Brix TH, Hegedüs L. Excess mortality in hyperthyroidism: The influence of preexisting comorbidity and genetic confounding: A Danish nationwide register-based cohort study of twins and singletons. The Journal of Clinical Endocrinology and Metabolism. 2012;**97**(11):4123-4129

[10] Bhat MH, Bhat JA, Masoodi SR, Qureshi W, Dar JR, Bhat MH. Clinical spectrum and outcome of patients with Graves' disease: A single-center experience from a tertiary care institution in the Kashmir Valley, India. Turkish Journal of Endocrinology and Metabolism. 2021;**25**(1):21-31

[11] Sundaresh V, Brito JP, Thapa P, Bahn RS, Stan MN. Comparative effectiveness of treatment choices for graves' hyperthyroidism: A historical cohort study. Thyroid The Official Journal of: American Thyroid Association. 2017;**27**(4):497-505

[12] Emiliano AB, Governale L, Parks M, Cooper DS. Shifts in propylthiouracil and methimazole prescribing practices: Antithyroid drug use in the United States from 1991 to 2008. The Journal of Clinical Endocrinology and Metabolism. 2010;**95**(5):2227-2233

[13] Ahad F, Ganie SA. Iodine, iodine metabolism and iodine deficiency disorders revisited. Indian Journal of Endocrinology and Metabolism. 2010;**14**(1):13-17

[14] Cooper DS. Antithyroid drugs in the management of patients with Graves' disease: An evidence-based approach to therapeutic controversies. The Journal of Clinical Endocrinology and Metabolism. 2003;**88**(8):3474-3481

[15] Abraham P, Acharya S. Current and emerging treatment options for Graves'

hyperthyroidism. Therapeutics and Clinical Risk Management. 2010;**6**:29-40

[16] Ross DS, Burch HB, Cooper DS, Greenlee MC, Laurberg P, Maia AL, et al. 2016 American thyroid association guidelines for diagnosis and management of hyperthyroidism and other causes of thyrotoxicosis. Thyroid The Official Journal of: American Thyroid Association. 2016;**26**(10):1343-1421

[17] Cooper DS. Antithyroid drugs. The New England Journal of Medicine. 2005;**352**(9):905-917

[18] Jansson R, Lindström B, Dahlberg PA. Pharmacokinetic properties and bioavailability of methimazole. Clinical Pharmacokinetics. 1985;**10**(5):443-450

[19] Jansson R, Dahlberg PA, Johansson H, Lindström B. Intrathyroidal concentrations of methimazole in patients with Graves' disease. The Journal of Clinical Endocrinology and Metabolism. 1983;**57**(1):129-132

[20] Liu L, Lu H, Liu Y, Liu C, Xun C. Predicting relapse of Graves' disease following treatment with antithyroid drugs. Experimental and Therapeutic Medicine. 2016;**11**(4):1453-1458

[21] MacFarlane IA, Davies D, Longson D, Shalet SM, Beardwell CG. Single daily dose short term carbimazole therapy for hyperthyroid Graves' disease. Clinical Endocrinology. 1983;**18**(6):557-561

[22] Gupta SK, Mithal A, Godbole MM. Single daily dose of carbimazole in the treatment of hyperthyroidism. National Medical Journal of India. 1992;**5**(5):214-216

[23] Idrose AM. Acute and emergency care for thyrotoxicosis and thyroid storm. Acute Medicine & Surgery. 2015;**2**(3):147-157

[24] Yu W, Wu N, Li L, Wang J, OuYang H, Shen H. Side effects of PTU and MMI in the treatment of hyperthyroidism: A systematic review and meta-analysis. Endocrine Practice of Official Journal of American College of Endocrinology and American Association of Clinical Endocrinologists. 2020;**26**(2):207-217

[25] Nicholas WC, Fischer RG, Stevenson RA, Bass JD. Single daily dose of methimazole compared to every 8 hours propylthiouracil in the treatment of hyperthyroidism. Southern Medical Journal. 1995;**88**(9):973-976

[26] Abbara A, Clarke SA, Brewster R, Simonnard A, Eng PC, Phylactou M, et al. Pharmacodynamic response to anti-thyroid drugs in Graves' hyperthyroidism. Frontiers in Endocrinology. 2020;**11**:286

[27] Bartalena L. Diagnosis and management of Graves disease: A global overview. Nature Reviews. Endocrinology. 2013;**9**(12):724-734

[28] Nakamura H, Noh JY, Itoh K, Fukata S, Miyauchi A, Hamada N. Comparison of methimazole and propylthiouracil in patients with hyperthyroidism caused by Graves' disease. The Journal of Clinical Endocrinology and Metabolism. 2007;**92**(6):2157-2162

[29] Vasileiou M, Gilbert J, Fishburn S, Boelaert K. Thyroid disease assessment and management: Summary of NICE guidance. British Medical Journal. 2020;**368**:m41

[30] Pouget JP, Lozza C, Deshayes E, Boudousq V, Navarro-Teulon I. Introduction to radiobiology of targeted radionuclide therapy. Frontiers in Medicine. 2015;**2**:12

[31] Metso S, Jaatinen P, Huhtala H, Luukkaala T, Oksala H, Salmi J.

Long-term follow-up study of radioiodine treatment of hyperthyroidism. Clinical Endocrinology. 2004;**61**(5):641-648

[32] Tran P, Desimone S, Barrett M, Bachrach B. I-131 treatment of graves' disease in an unsuspected first trimester pregnancy; the potential for adverse effects on the fetus and a review of the current guidelines for pregnancy screening. International Journal of Pediatric Endocrinology. 2010;**2010**:858359

[33] Stokkel MPM, Handkiewicz Junak D, Lassmann M, Dietlein M, Luster M. EANM procedure guidelines for therapy of benign thyroid disease. European Journal of Nuclear Medicine and Molecular Imaging. 2010;**37**(11):2218-2228

[34] Andrade VA, Gross JL, Maia AL. The effect of methimazole pretreatment on the efficacy of radioactive iodine therapy in Graves' hyperthyroidism: One-year follow-up of a prospective, randomized study. The Journal of Clinical Endocrinology and Metabolism. 2001;**86**(8):3488-3493

[35] Rivkees SA, Sklar C, Freemark M. Clinical review 99: The management of Graves' disease in children, with special emphasis on radioiodine treatment. The Journal of Clinical Endocrinology and Metabolism. 1998;**83**(11):3767-3776

[36] Törring O, Tallstedt L, Wallin G, Lundell G, Ljunggren JG, Taube A, et al. Graves' hyperthyroidism: Treatment with antithyroid drugs, surgery, or radioiodine–a prospective, randomized study. Thyroid Study Group. The Journal of Clinical Endocrinology and Metabolism. 1996;**81**(8):2986-2993

[37] Feroci F, Rettori M, Borrelli A, Coppola A, Castagnoli A, Perigli G, et al. A systematic review and meta-analysis of total thyroidectomy versus bilateral subtotal thyroidectomy for Graves' disease. Surgery. 2014;**155**(3):529-540

[38] Smithson M, Asban A, Miller J, Chen H. Considerations for thyroidectomy as treatment for Graves disease. Clinical Medicine Insights: Endocrinology and Diabetes. 2019;**12**:1179551419844523

[39] Barczyński M, Konturek A, Hubalewska-Dydejczyk A, Gołkowski F, Nowak W. Randomized clinical trial of bilateral subtotal thyroidectomy versus total thyroidectomy for Graves' disease with a 5-year follow-up. The British Journal of Surgery. 2012;**99**(4):515-522

[40] Bahn Chair RS, Burch HB, Cooper DS, Garber JR, Greenlee MC, Klein I, et al. Hyperthyroidism and other causes of thyrotoxicosis: Management guidelines of the american thyroid association and American association of clinical endocrinologists. Thyroid The Official Journal of: American Thyroid Association. 2011;**21**(6):593-646

[41] Robert J, Mariéthoz S, Pache JC, Bertin D, Caulfield A, Murith N, et al. Short- and long-term results of total vs subtotal thyroidectomies in the surgical treatment of Graves' disease. Swiss Surgery Schweizer Chirurgie Chirurgie Suisse Chirurgia Svizzera. 2001;**7**(1):20-24

[42] Werga-Kjellman P, Zedenius J, Tallstedt L, Träisk F, Lundell G, Wallin G. Surgical treatment of hyperthyroidism: A ten-year experience. Thyroid The Official Journal of: American Thyroid Association. 2001;**11**(2):187-192

[43] Lepner U, Seire I, Palmiste V, Kirsimägi U. Surgical treatment of Graves' disease: Subtotal thyroidectomy might still be the preferred option. Medicina (Kaunas, Lithuania). 2008;**44**(1):22-26

[44] Cooper DS, Laurberg P. Hyperthyroidism in pregnancy. The Lancet Diabetes and Endocrinology. 2013;**1**(3):238-249

[45] Andersen SL, Olsen J, Laurberg P. Antithyroid drug side effects in the population and in pregnancy. The Journal of Clinical Endocrinology and Metabolism. 2016;**101**(4):1606-1614

[46] Momotani N, Yamashita R, Makino F, Noh JY, Ishikawa N, Ito K. Thyroid function in wholly breast-feeding infants whose mothers take high doses of propylthiouracil. Clinical Endocrinology. 2000;**53**(2):177-181

[47] Azizi F, Khoshniat M, Bahrainian M, Hedayati M. Thyroid function and intellectual development of infants nursed by mothers taking methimazole. The Journal of Clinical Endocrinology and Metabolism. 2000;**85**(9):3233-3238

[48] Mandel SJ, Cooper DS. The use of antithyroid drugs in pregnancy and lactation. The Journal of Clinical Endocrinology and Metabolism. 2001;**86**(6):2354-2359

[49] Abalovich M, Amino N, Barbour LA, Cobin RH, De Groot LJ, Glinoer D, et al. Management of thyroid dysfunction during pregnancy and postpartum: An endocrine society clinical practice guideline. The Journal of Clinical Endocrinology and Metabolism. 2007;**92**(8 Suppl):S1-S47

[50] Pearce SHS, Dayan C, Wraith DC, Barrell K, Olive N, Jansson L, et al. Antigen-specific immunotherapy with thyrotropin receptor peptides in graves' hyperthyroidism: A phase I study. Thyroid. 2019;**29**(7):1003-1011

[51] Lane LC, Cheetham TD, Perros P, Pearce SHS. New therapeutic horizons for graves' hyperthyroidism. Endocrine Reviews. 2020;**41**(6):bnaa022

Section 4

Diseases Associated with Hyperthyroidism

Chapter 5

The Impact of Hyperthyroidism on Fertility, Maternal, Foetal and Perinatal Outcomes in the Era of Iodine Fortification

Constance Nontsikelelo Gubu-Ntaba, Vulikhaya Mpumlwana, Nandipha Mizpa Sotobe-Mbana, Martha Mayer, Chukwuma Ogbonna Ekpebegh and Charles Bitamazire Businge

Abstract

Graves' disease and nodular toxic thyroid disease are the leading causes of hyperthyroidism. Iodine fortification (IF) among mild-to-moderate iodine deficiency populations is associated with transient increase in incident thyrotoxic nodular disease that may last up to 10 years. A rise in incident Graves' disease and other autoimmune thyroid conditions has also been associated with IF. Epidemiological studies from different geographical settings around the globe suggest increased incidence even among reproductive age groups in affected populations. Recurrent iodine deficiency in iodine replete populations in developed countries may also predispose them to a similar phenomenon. The prevalence and consequences of hyperthyroidism in pregnancy may be higher than previously reported. We intend to describe the aetiopathology and epidemiology of hyperthyroidism, the mechanisms through which hyperthyroidism predisposes to infertility; the impact of hyperthyroidism on fertility treatment, pregnancy in general and among women with infertility; as well as the effects of hyperthyroidism or agents used in the treatment of hyperthyroidism on perinatal outcomes and adult life for those exposed *in utero*.

Keywords: hyperthyroidism, infertility, maternal and neonatal outcomes, antithyroid drugs, iodine fortification

1. Introduction

Thyroid hormones control the metabolism of all nucleated cells and hence are vital for the various processes involved in gametogenesis, fertilisation, embryogenesis, implantation, foetal development and growth *in utero* [1, 2]. Hyperthyroidism is a pathological state characterised by excessive production of thyroid hormones and subsequent elevation of serum levels of thyroxine (T4) and triiodothyronine (T3) and diminution of serum thyroid-stimulating hormone levels [3]. The different aetio-pathological mechanisms leading to hyperthyroidism as well as the various treatment modalities can potentially have a negative impact on male and female fertility, conception, foetal and maternal well-being, as well perinatal and adult life of foetuses exposed *in utero* [2, 4, 5]. Previously hyperthyroidism was reported as having a low prevalence of less than 1%, mainly affecting middle-aged and elderly populations [6]. Recent epidemiological surveys suggest the prevalence rates of up to 1.6% in populations recovering from endemic iodine deficiency following universal iodisation of salt, mainly presenting as toxic thyroid nodules, not only among the elderly but including persons in the age range 20–49 years [7–9]. Pedersen et al. [7] reported an increase of prevalence of hyperthyroidism of 160% in the 20–39 age group in Denmark following food fortification with iodine. In Ghana, following 20 years of universal iodization of salt, Sarfo-Kantanka et al. [8] reported an increase in the incidence of thyroid diseases-related hospital admissions 213 to 538/100,00 admissions. Toxic nodular goitre was the second most common presentation with a percentage of 22.5%, affecting mainly women (female: male ratio of 8.3:1) age range of 27–42 years. This increase in hyperthyroidism following improved access to iodine nutrition although transient but can last up to 10 years [10, 11]. This is followed by a decline in the prevalence of hyperthyroidism in countries that attain and maintain optimal iodine nutrition [7, 9, 12]. It is not clear whether excessive iodine intake in formerly iodine deficiency endemic populations, or recurrent exposure to iodine deficiency in pregnancy like, has been reported in some European countries [13, 14] can lead to prolong the 'transient increase' in hyperthyroidism secondary to iodine fortification. One study from south China reported that pregnancy not only predisposes to hypertrophy of pre-existing nodules, also but to the formation of new nodules with biochemical milieu close to subclinical hyperthyroidism [15].

Some of the increase in prevalence of hyperthyroidism among younger people following fortification of food with iodine has been attributed to thyroid autoimmune disorders. This is in addition to thyroid nodules that were previously reported to be more common among middle aged and the elderly populations that are also increasingly prevalent among people in reproductive years [10, 16]. Graves' disease that has been traditionally reported to be more prevalent in developed iodine-sufficient countries has also been reported in recent studies done in countries recovering from endemic iodine deficiency [17]. This has in part been attributed to an epidemiological transition, or better diagnostic capacity in recent times with many cases remaining undiagnosed in the past.

With an estimated 1.88 billion people at risk of mild-to-moderate iodine deficiency in both developed and developing world and concerted effort to improve iodine nutrition through food fortification [18, 19], the incidence of transient hyperthyroidism at population level secondary to improved iodine nutrition is likely to lead to higher prevalence of hyperthyroidism secondary to nodular thyroid and Graves' disease. Hence, the incidence of hyperthyroidism in developing both developing and developed countries undergoing iodine supplementation due to endemic or recurrent mild-to-moderate iodine deficiency may be higher than previously reported. This not only requires a better understanding of the effect of hyperthyroidism on pregnancy, but also on fertility, and on neonatal and adult life of those exposed to hyperthyroidism and various treatments *in utero*.

In this chapter we intend to

- Describe the aetiopathology and epidemiology of hyperthyroidism

- Outline the mechanisms through which hyperthyroidism may predispose to infertility
- Explore the impact of hyperthyroidism on fertility treatment
- Explore the impact of hyperthyroidism on foetal and maternal well-being
- Highlight the impact of hyperthyroidism on post-partum maternal health, perinatal and childhood and adult life of children exposed *in utero*

2. Aetiology and pathogenesis

Hyperthyroidism has a female predilection (sex ratio of 5:1), and a life time risk of 2–5% with a modal age of presentation among females is 20 and 40 years [20]. More than 99% of all patients with hyperthyroidism are as a result of pathological processes within the thyroid gland leading to hyperactivity and excessive secretion of T3 and T4 [20]. Excessive secretion of TSH from the pituitary is an uncommon cause.

Graves' disease, an autoimmune disorder in which stimulatory serum IgG antibodies bind to TSH receptors in the thyroid leading to excessive output of T3 and T4 secretion from the thyroid gland into the circulation, is the leading cause in iodine-sufficient regions of the world [20]. Graves' disease tends to affect the young- and middle-aged people [20, 21] and it thought to result from molecular mimicry following infection with bacteria such as *Escherichia coli* and *Yersinia enterocolitica* that possess TSH-binding sites [22]. Other risk factors of Graves' disease include HLA-mediated genetic predisposition as well as smoking [20, 23].

Toxic nodular thyroid lesions are the second most frequent cause of hyperthyroidism and the leading cause in iodine-deficient areas [24]. Previously, toxic thyroid disease associated with iodine deficient was reported to be more prevalent in the elderly [25]. The aetiology of thyroid glandular lesions leading to hyperthyroidism is related to the degree of iodine nutrition of the population [26]. Following the implementation of universal iodization of salt (USI) globally, studies from formerly iodine deficiency endemic areas reported an increased incidence of both Graves' disease and toxic nodular thyroid disease also affecting not only the elderly populations, but also segments of the population in the reproductive age [8, 9, 11]. Like Graves' disease, females are more prone to solitary toxic nodules than males with F:M ratio > 4.8 [8]. Toxic nodular thyroid disease compared to Graves' disease is more prone to resurgence of thyrotoxicosis after achieving euthyroid state with antithyroid drugs [27].

Among populations with low levels of dietary iodine intake, the thyroid gland tries to ensure adequate hormonal production through increased activity of the thyroid follicular cells. Prolongation of this compensatory hyperactivity due to persistent iodine deficiency results into autonomous growth and function of clusters of follicular cells [25]. The increase in dietary iodine intake following the advent of USI implemented in various countries with low-to-moderate severe iodine deficiency results in excessive output of thyroid hormones from the autonomous follicular clusters resulting into nodular toxic thyrotoxicosis [26]. This increased incidence in hyperthyroidism including people of reproductive age requires a concerted effort aimed at preconception diagnosis and management of hyperthyroid disease in people of reproductive age and in early pregnancy so as to mitigate the short- and long-term foetal, perinatal, maternal and adult life complications associated with uncontrolled hyperthyroidism and its treatment.

Gestational hyperthyroidism also known as gestational transient thyrotoxicosis (GTT) is a transient elevation of serum thyroid hormone levels in pregnant women without evidence of thyroid autoimmunity. GTT affects 1–5% of pregnant women early in pregnancy. This form of thyrotoxicosis usually resolves spontaneously by the end of the first or early second trimester of pregnancy. This is attributed to the physiological elevation of serum HCG, which peaks in the first 8 to 11 weeks of pregnancy, decreasing thereafter, and remaining in plateau up to term [28–31]. GTT has a short and self-limiting course and does not usually require specific treatment. Milder forms are likely to remain unrecognised. Free T4 levels tend to return to normal in the second trimester; hence, supportive management is generally all that is needed [4]. However, in severe form GTT presents as hyperemesis gravidarum, with significant weight loss and thyrotoxicotic features such as tachycardia, hyperreflexia, hand tremors but without goitre or orbitopathy usually associated with Graves' disease [4].

3. Differential diagnosis

Differential diagnoses of hyperthyroidism are conditions that predispose to thyrotoxicosis without intrinsic hyperactivity of the thyroid gland. These include thyroid pathology that leads to destruction of the follicular cells and consequential release of the preformed T3 and T4 leading to transient thyrotoxicosis. Examples include post-partum thyroiditis, silent thyroiditis and sub-acute painful thyroiditis. Others include iatrogenic T4 administration, medications such as lithium, interferon α and amiodarone, as well as metastatic thyroid carcinoma and thyroid hormone-producing tumours such as struma ovarii [3] and trophoblastic diseases that produce excessive β-HCG that is not only structurally similar to thyroid-stimulating hormone but has accentuated stimulation of the thyroid follicular cells than the normal hCG [32].

4. Hyperthyroidism and reproduction

Thyroid dysfunction is the most commonly found endocrine problem in females of reproductive age [33]. Hyperthyroidism (both clinical and subclinical) can affect both males and females of reproductive age, by producing variable degrees of gonadal dysfunction [33, 34]. In the general population, it affects 1.5% of reproductive age females and 2.3% of the infertile group [35]. It is associated with infertility, though this is not well established due to limited evidence [36]. According to WHO, infertility is failure to achieve successful pregnancy after 12 months or more of appropriate, timed, unprotected intercourse [37]. Although there is no evidence of improved ovulation rates, treatment of both clinical and subclinical hyperthyroidism is advisable to improve pregnancy adverse outcomes, including early pregnancy loss [35, 36].

4.1 Effect of hyperthyroidism on the hypothalamic, pituitary gonadal axis

Thyrotoxicosis in females is associated with increased GnRH sensitivity, though most women will still have ovulatory cycles [36, 37]. Other hormonal changes in a female include an increase in the production of sex hormone-binding globulin

(SHBG) and oestrogen with decreased oestrogen clearance. Thyrotoxicosis is also associated with the increased production of androgens such as androstenedione and testosterone that are subsequently converted to estrone [34, 38].

Hyperthyroidism is associated with delayed puberty [32]. Post-puberty hyperthyroidism may be associated with hypomenorrhea, polymenorrhea, oligomenorrhea and hypermenorrhea [34]. These menstrual disturbances are found in about 22% of women with hyperthyroidism compared to 8% of healthy controls [39].

Hyperthyroidism in males is associated with increased incidence of gynecomastia, as well as decreased libido which is attributed to increased levels of free oestrogen [34]. Hyperthyroidism causes oligozoospermia, asthenozoospermia and teratozoospermia, the mechanisms by which these adverse effects come about is poorly understood [40].

4.2 Autoimmune thyroid disease (AITD) and fertility

Thyroid autoimmune is present in up to 25% of the general population [35]. AITD is associated with poor outcomes pregnancy outcomes among women in reproductive age who are euthyroid, especially those who are undergoing assisted reproduction [35]. The thyroid is affected by autoimmune disease *via* T cells, commonly causing to Graves' disease and Hashimoto's thyroiditis accompanied with hyperthyroidism or hypothyroidism [30]. Most common antibodies include thyroid peroxidase antibodies, thyroglobulin antibodies and thyroid-stimulating hormone receptor antibodies. Thyroid-stimulating antibodies are central to the pathogenesis of Graves' disease, while other antibodies are produced as a response to thyroid injury leading to hypothyroidism. Thyroid-stimulating antibodies have a limited effect on fertility, but have a role in foetal and neonatal hyperthyroidism [30].

The radioactive iodine treatment commonly used for hyperthyroidism, especially Grave's disease does not have an effect on gonadal function but pregnancy should be postponed by at least 6 months after treatment because of teratogenic effect [31, 35].

5. Preconception care

The best maternal and prenatal outcomes are expected from women who are healthy at the onset of pregnancy [41]. Pregnancy among women with hyperthyroidism faces a two-pronged challenge: potential complications from metabolic derangements secondary to excessive thyroid hormones and circulating auto-antibodies among women with Graves' disease; and the adverse effects of the varied treatment remedies aimed at the control thyroid function close to the normal state [4]. The principles of preconception care for women with hyperthyroidism are to use effective contraception until the patient achieves a sustained euthyroid state [42]. This will reduce the complications associated with the deranged metabolic state due to excessive thyroid hormones in the circulation.

In order to reduce the risk of teratogenicity, women who have attained a euthyroid state preconceptionally when treated with carbimazole or methimazole should be switched to propylthiouracil till a stable euthyroid state is maintained before attempting to conceive [43]. Treatment with propylthiouracil should be continued until organogenesis is deemed complete at the end of the first trimester.

Since pregnancy is associated with diminution of cell-mediated immunity and reduced risk of relapse, an alternative strategy for euthyroid women with Graves' disease with TSH receptor antibodies (TRab) below cut-off level, on minimum doses of antithyroid drugs is to withhold the antithyroid drugs at the inception of pregnancy. Then, they are to be followed closely with prompt reinstatement of treatment in case of relapse [43, 44]. Women who still desire pregnancy but are at high risk of relapse due to high-circulating levels of TRab titres should be counselled for the option of total thyroidectomy and thyroid hormone replacement [44].

6. Thyroid physiology in pregnancy

The thyroid gland produces T3 and T4 which are essential for normal maternal and foetal metabolism. The hypothalamic-pituitary-thyroid axis is important for this control [45]. Increase in oestrogen concentration in pregnancy results in elevated hepatic synthesis of thyroid-binding globulin (TBG) necessitating increased T3and T4 output from the thyroid gland. This coupled with relative iodine deficiency due to increased maternal glomerular excretion, and transplacental transfer of iodine to the foetus combined with high levels of HCG leads to maternal thyroid hyperstimulation [46]. This increases the serum T4 and T3 levels between 6 and 12 weeks of gestation reaching a plateau at 20 weeks which through negative feedback reduces TSH secretion from the pituitary [46, 47]. In early pregnancy, there is transplacental transfer of maternal T4 but not TSH which is essential for foetal metabolism and normal neurological development. In the second trimester, there is placental metabolism of maternal thyroid hormones and the foetal thyroid takes over thyroid hormone synthesis using iodine obtained through transplacental transfer from the mother [29].

The normal range of thyroid function tests in pregnancy varies according to iodine dietary content and ethnicity, and fluctuations across the trimesters of pregnancy [48]. Total T4 (tT4) has been found to be more reliable for measurement during pregnancy compared with fT3 and fT4. To adjust for the general increase of tT4 in pregnancy compared to non-pregnancy state, it is recommended that the levels should be multiplied by 1.5. As an option fT4 index may also be used in pregnancy, as it corrects tT4 according to the TBG levels [48].

6.1 Hyperthyroidism and interpretation of results in pregnancy

HCG, which is structurally similar to TSH molecule, has a weak stimulatory effect on the thyroid cells resulting in elevated T4 and T3 [28, 29]. A negative feedback effect of the elevated thyroid hormones on the anterior pituitary results in low levels of TSH [48]. This reduction is estimated to be about 0.1–0.2 mU/L for the lower limit and 0.5–1.0 mU/L for the upper limit compared to non-pregnant state [41]. HCG levels decrease in the second trimester; therefore, TSH level rises again [48]. The use of trimester-specific TSH reference values is necessary in pregnancy due to these physiological changes that result in modification of the normal reference ranges of serum thyroid-stimulating hormone. Free serum T4 (FT4) estimates are unreliable during pregnancy compared to TSH that remains sensitive in pregnancy despite the effects of HCG (human chorionic gonadotropin) (**Table 1**) [41].

6.2 Clinical features of hyperthyroidism pregnancy

The clinical features of hyperthyroidism overlap with those of pregnancy and hence may make diagnosis difficult especially for a patient who develops incident

Test	Non-pregnant state	First trimester	Second trimester	Third trimester
TSH	0.3–4.2	0.1–2.5 mIU/L	0.2–3.0 mlU/l	0.3–3.0mlU/L
fT4 (pmol/l)	9.0–26.0	10-16 pmol/l	9.5–15.5 pmol/l	8–14.5 pmol/l
fT3 (pmol/l)	2.6–5.7	3-7 pmol/l	3–5.5 pmol/l	2.5–5.5 pmol/l
Refs. [41, 48].				

Table 1.
Comparison of serum thyroid hormone levels in pregnancy and non-pregnant state.

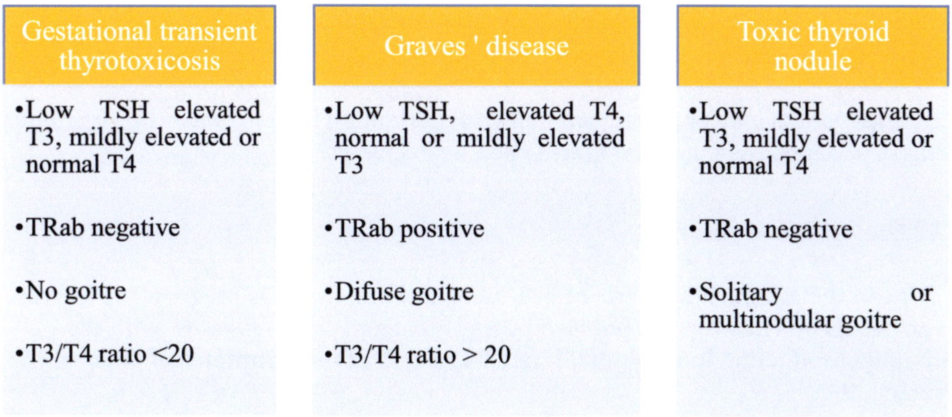

Figure 1.
Biochemical features of gestational thyrotoxicosis, Graves' disease and nodular thyroid disease.

hyperthyroidism in the first trimester of pregnancy [49]. These include palpitations dyspnoea, fatigue, sweating and haemic murmurs. If these features become severe in addition to nervousness and hyperactivity, it is prudent to exclude thyrotoxicosis with its underlying cause.

Although graves' disease has traditionally been reported in the young adults, and nodular toxic thyrotoxicosis in older people, it is worthwhile to consider both conditions in addition to gestational thyrotoxicosis when presented with a symptomatic pregnant woman [10, 16]. This is informed by the increased prevalence of both autoimmune and nodular thyroid disease with iodine fortification coupled with recurrent migration within and between countries and continents [15].

Some features that can help distinguish between the three commonest underlying causes of thyrotoxicosis in pregnancy are shown in **Figure 1** and **Table 2** [50–52].

6.3 Effect of pregnancy on the common underlying entities of thyrotoxicosis

6.3.1 GTT

Since gestational transient thyrotoxicosis is caused by excessive hCG or in heritable TSHR hypersensitivity to hCG, GTT will be self-limiting and most patients will revert to normal thyroid function after the first trimester especially by about 20-week gestation following the natural reduction in serum hCG [51]. However, thyrotoxicosis may persist beyond the first trimester among women with hyper-placentosis such as

Clinical features	GD	GTT	TMG &TA
Symptoms pre-dating pregnancy	++	—	+/−
Symptoms during pregnancy	+/+++	+/−	+/−
Nausea/vomiting	−/+	+++++	+/−
Persistence of symptoms	May subside	Subsides in second half	May worsen
Goitre	+	—	+
Orbitopathy	+	—	—

Table 2.
Differentiating clinical features of Graves' disease, gestational thyrotoxicosis and toxic nodular disease.

in multiple pregnancy or among women with heritable TSHR hypersensitivity to hCG. In these patients, toxic nodular goitre need be excluded.

6.3.2 Graves' disease

Due to the diminishing levels of cell-mediated immunity as pregnancy progresses, serum levels of TRab tend to reduce in the second and third trimester with the consequent reduction in levels of T3 and T4 as well as the symptoms of Graves' disease [29].

6.3.3 Toxic thyroid nodules

Pregnancy is associated with increase in the size and number of thyroid nodules especially among women of higher parity [15]. This may potentially increase the severity of thyrotoxicosis and the necessity for treatment or increase in doses of ATD or lead to surgical intervention.

6.4 Impact of thyrotoxicosis on pregnancy

Without optimum maternal treatment, hyperthyroidism in pregnancy is associated with maternal and foetal adverse outcomes. This could be secondary to the high metabolic state and specific pathological processes, and ATD [29, 41].

6.4.1 Impact on maternal health

Severe GTT may be associated with hyperemesis gravidarum that in addition to features of thyrotoxicosis will present with weight loss of ≥5%, dehydration and ketonuria [4]. Rather than being a direct complication this may be due to the shared mechanism of high levels or hypersensitivity to circulating hCG.

Maternal nodular goitre can lead to tracheal obstruction. Irrespective of the primary cause, high levels of thyroid hormones T3 and T4 may predispose to maternal arrythmias and cardiac failure, or thyroid storm, miscarriage, abruptio placenta and preeclampsia. Elevated TRAb preconception is a prognostic of risk for relapse of GD, failing ATD or cessation [53].

6.4.2 Maternal complications

Maternal complications of hyperthyroidism include preeclampsia, abruptio placenta, incident diabetes mellitus, thyroid storm, and arrhythmia, congestive heart failure, and cardiovascular disease [4, 41]. In a recent systematic review and meta-analysis, Alves et al. [5] found that the treatment of hyperthyroidism was associated with reduced risk of abruptio placentae, gestational diabetes mellitus and postpartum haemorrhage.

6.5 Management of hyperthyroidism in pregnancy

Optimum management of hyperthyroidism in pregnancy necessitated a multidisciplinary team comprising of an obstetrician, maternal foetal medicine specialist and paediatric endocrinologist, and a neonatologist is necessary, and sometimes adult and paediatric critical care specialists if complications arise [29]. The aim of treatment is to achieve near-euthyroid state without causing adverse effects to the mother and the foetus.

Challenges of treatment include the following:

- Radioiodine crosses the placenta leading to foetal thyroid ablation so is contraindicated in pregnancy.

- Surgery predisposes to pregnancy losses especially in first and third trimester and severe haemorrhage and laryngeal nerve injury to the mother so it is best differed to post-partum period or if unavoidable done in the second trimester [45, 54].

- ATDs cross the placenta, predispose to congenital defects if used in the first trimester, and in high doses predispose to foetal hypothyroidism.

6.5.1 Management of GTT

GTT is usually self-limiting hence symptomatic treatment is usually recommended [49]. If symptoms persist beyond 16 weeks gestation into the second half of pregnancy, or is severe enough to require ATD, the patient should be re-valuated and screened for GD, toxic adenoma or TMN goitre.

6.5.2 Management of thyrotoxicosis among women with GD, toxic adenoma and multinodular goitre in pregnancy

The management includes administration of ATD, beta-blockers and supportive treatment as needed. The mechanism of action of thionamides is to block the synthesis of thyroid hormones; in addition, PTU blocks the peripheral conversion of T4 to more potent T3 [55]. The aim of ATD therapy is to maintain thyroid hormones levels at the upper point of the normal range with the minimum possible dosages of the drugs. PTU should be used in the first trimester as recommended and then later substituted with methimazole in the second trimester to avoid hepatotoxicity associated with it. Adjunctive treatment with beta-adrenergic blockers may be used to reduce tachycardia, palpitations and tremors. Propranolol 20 to 40 mg orally every 8 to 12 hours may be used while awaiting response to the antithyroid medications [4]. Antithyroid medications can and should be tapered as pregnancy progresses [56]. When serum TSH rises to detectable level, this is an indication to reduce ATD.

In patients in with GD in which ATD is discontinued in the third trimester, close monitoring should be done in the postpartum period due to high risk of relapse [56]. The indications for thyroidectomy include severe thyrotoxic orbitopathy, high TRab titres post-radioiodine therapy in GD, obstructive goitre and adverse drug reaction [54].

Since the risk of recurrence of toxic multinodular goitre treated with ATD is more than 95%, patients with thyrotoxic multinodular disease treated with ATD during pregnancy should be considered for thyroidectomy in the in the postpartum period [27].

7. Maternal hyperthyroidism and the foetus

The foetal thyroid gland develops 24-days post-conception and is capable of taking up iodine from 10 to 11 weeks. Foetal thyroid hormone production is controlled by the foetal hypothalamo-pituitary axis beginning 20 weeks after conception. Foetal levels of TSH, T4 and T3 reach adult levels by 36 weeks [55]. Transplacental passage of maternal thyroid-stimulating antibodies or ATD, both of which may disrupt foetal thyroid function have an effect on foetal prognosis [29].

7.1 Effect of TRab on the foetus

The foetus may develop thyrotoxicosis secondary to the maternal receptor antibodies, which having crossed the placenta stimulates the adenylate cyclase in foetal thyrocytes. The foetus of untreated or mothers with poorly controlled GD disease may be complicated by foetal goitre, intrauterine growth retardation, low birth weight and preterm birth or foetal death may occur [4]. These foetal complications have also been observed in pregnancies of some women with Graves' disease that became euthyroid after surgical or radioiodine treatment that remained with high-serum thyroid receptor antibodies [57]. The detection of TRAbs in pregnancy should result in the foetus being considered at risk of developing thyrotoxicosis and monitored accordingly [58].

7.2 Effects of maternal ATD therapy on the foetal thyroid

All available ATDs (MMI, CM, PTU) cross the placenta and therefore have the potential to cause foetal hypothyroidism [4]. Early exposure in pregnancy to ATD has been associated with birth defects [4]. PTU is associated with less common and less severe teratogenicity than MMI (**Table 3**) [59]. ATD doses necessary to maintain maternal FT4 in the upper normal to mildly thyrotoxic range are associated with normal foetal thyroid function. Higher doses of ATD predispose to foetal hypothyroidism and goitre [4]. Therefore, it is recommended the lowest effective dose of MMI or PTU to maintain maternal serum FT4/TT4 at or moderately above the upper limit of the reference range should be used.

The 'Block' and 'replace' treatment method with ATD and levothyroxine (LT4) should be avoided in pregnancy because the transplacental passage of ATD is high, whereas it is negligible for thyroid hormones; hence, addition of LT4 will not protect the foetus from ATD-induced hypothyroidism [60, 61].

Carbimazole/methimazole	PTU
Aplasia cutis	Pre-auricular sinus/fistula and cysts
Choanal/oesophageal atresia	Urinary tract abnormalities in males
Hearing loss	
Dysmorphic features	
Developmental delay	
Omphalocele	
Omphalomesenteric duct abnormalities	
Refs. [4, 59].	

Table 3.
Birth defects associated with ATDs.

7.3 Foetal ultrasound

Mothers with positive Trab should be referred to a maternal foetal medicine specialist for foetal surveillance. This includes foetal ultrasound in the first trimester for dating and nuchal translucency (NT scan), foetal anomaly scan at 18–22 weeks and 2–3 weekly scans to screen for adverse effects of TRab and ATD. Ultrasound features of foetal hyperthyroidism include goitre detected as a solid hyperechogenic vascular neck mass [60], tachycardia, hydrops, polyhydramnios and risk of premature rupture of membranes and preterm labour and foetal growth restriction [4].

Foetal hypothyroidism may be diagnosed by the presence of a large goitre, polyhydramnios and bradycardia. Demonstration of peripheral blood flow on foetal thyroid Doppler ultrasound differentiates goitre due to foetal hypothyroidism from that due to foetal hyperthyroidism, which has both peripheral and central blood flow [62].

7.4 Management of foetal complications

The mainstay of treatment of foetal GD secondary to transplacental maternal TRab regardless of maternal thyroid state is the administration of ATD to the mother and monitoring of reduction of foetal goitre and foetal heart rate. In case maternal hypothyroidism ensues, this is managed with levothyroxine replacement [41].

The approach to foetal hypothyroidism secondary to maternal ATD is to reduce the dose and aim to keep the T4 levels closer to the upper limit of normal [52]. In rare cases where hypothyroidism does not resolve following reduction of maternal ATD doses, invasive therapy with intra-amniotic levothyroxine at a dose of 10mcg/kg/week for several weeks can be given [52].

When foetal goitre persists to time of delivery a planned elective caesarean section should be performed with EX-Utero Intrapartum Treatment (EXIT) procedure to secure the airway with intubation while still maintaining placental circulation [60].

8. Children Born to Mothers with Hyperthyroidism

Since GTT is usually self-limiting [29], children born to mothers with GTT are expected to be healthy at birth. Those born to mothers with Graves and nodular thyrotoxicosis requiring treatment may present with complications secondary to transplacental transfer of ATD [63]. Antithyroid drugs are also transferred into the breast milk and this has been previously thought to put the nursing neonate at risk of hypothyroidism. However, several studies evaluate thyroid function in infants whose mothers breastfed while taking PTU or MMI failed to detect the adverse effects on the newborn [64]. Continuation of breastfeeding is generally now considered safe and should be encouraged in hyperthyroid mothers taking ATD.

About 1–2% of neonates born to mothers with GD develop neonatal hyperthyroidism although some have reported an incidence as high as 5% [65, 66]. Neonatal thyrotoxicosis carries significant morbidity and mortality. In most cases, neonatal thyrotoxicosis is transient and results from the transplacental passage of maternal stimulating TSH receptor antibodies (TRAb) [66, 67]. TRAb may also be transferred to the baby by way of breastmilk and cause neonatal hyperthyroidism, which requires treatment even if the mother is euthyroid [67].

All infants born to mothers with a history of Graves' disease should undergo careful examination and monitoring to screen for the development of clinical hyperthyroidism and serious complications associated with it [29]. Neonates born to mothers with Graves' disease with good control on ATD may not have obvious symptoms of hyperthyroidism at birth, which may result in delayed diagnosis and complications [4]. Neonates born to mothers who tested negative for TRAb during the second half of gestation or those that exhibited absence of TRAb in the cord blood are unlikely to develop hyperthyroidism and are considered low-risk patients [68]. However, all neonates of mothers with hyperthyroidism require a focused assessment at birth for potential complications.

8.1 Clinical presentation of neonatal hyperthyroidism

The time of onset and severity of symptoms of hyperthyroidism are variable. Neonates born to mothers who had high TRAb levels (more than three times the upper normal value) and who were not treated with ATDs can exhibit overt hyperthyroidism at birth, while neonates born to mothers treated with ATDs or neonates who receive maternal thyroid receptor blocking antibodies may have normal thyroid function or present with hypothyroidism at birth [69, 70]. Some neonates of mothers with GD on antithyroid medication may be born with the features of hypothyroidism and later after about 2–5 days of life may show signs of hyperthyroidism following subsequent metabolism and excretion of maternal ATDs from their circulation [71].

The neonatal hyperthyroidism may present with a thyroid storm marked by tachycardia, hypertension, hyperthermia, tremors, irritability, restlessness, sweating, difficulty in sleeping, tachypnoea, arrhythmia, supraventricular tachycardia and cardiac failure [72]. Neonates with thyrotoxicosis and cardiac failure have a high mortality rate of up to 20% if not timely and adequately treated [73].

Maternal TRab may remain in the infant circulation for from a month up to 3 months, most neonates with congenital hyperthyroidism respond to ATD therapy within 1–2 months [74]. However, there might be some long-term adverse effects on cognitive development even with the prompt treatment.

Others may present with features such as frontal bossing, triangular face, periorbital oedema, goitre, hyperactivity, failure to thrive despite excessive appetite, reduction in the subcutaneous adipose tissue [68]. The neonate may also present with non-specific clinical features such as diarrhoea, vomiting, fever, sweating, pulmonary hypertension, chylothorax, jaundice, hepatosplenomegaly, prolonged acrocyanosis and sialadenitis. Premature closure of cranial sutures (craniosynostosis) and subsequent microcephaly may be noted in severely affected infants [75].

8.2 Laboratory tests for neonates with hyperthyroidism

It is recommended that neonates born to mothers with TRAb antibodies as well as neonates with a known family history of genetic congenital hyperthyroidism should have their cord blood tested for the TRAb between days 3 and 5 after birth, then at 2 weeks and 3 months [68, 76]. Thyroid function tests performed on the cord blood before the third day of life in neonates tend to reflect intrauterine foetal thyroid status and are poor predictors of neonatal hyperthyroidism. Thyroid function tests start showing biochemical picture in the neonates with hyperthyroidism between days 3 and 15 following birth [77].

High-risk infants with normal initial testing should have repeat blood workup at days 10–14 days of life or when symptoms appear. Hyperthyroidism in the newborn is suggested by high T4 and T3 levels with low TSH (<0.9 mlU/L) [66]. Additional investigations to check for other organ malfunction include AST, ALT and direct bilirubin, blood sugar, and platelets, cardiac and thyroid ultrasonography as well as wrist and hand X-ray for assessment of bone maturation [66].

8.3 Management of neonates with hyperthyroidism

Treatment should be promptly initiated upon clinical and biochemical diagnosis of neonatal hyperthyroidism [76]. Early and appropriate treatment is necessary in order to reduce the risk of heart failure in the acute phase. Adequate hydration should be maintained and airway, breathing and circulatory support should be provided if required [71]. Pharmacological treatment includes adrenergic blockage, inhibition thyroid hormone synthesis, release and peripheral conversion, reduction of preload afterload and regulation of cardiac rhythm and other supportive treatment (**Table 4**) [71]. Infants with persistent hyperthyroidism despite adequate medical treatment may require thyroidectomy [66].

8.4 Pathogenesis of congenital hypothyroidism among neonates born to mothers with hyperthyroidism

Some neonates of mothers with hyperthyroidism may be born with congenital hypothyroidism which may be central or primary. Primary neonatal hypothyroidism may occur among children born to mothers on ATD, or Graves' disease secondary to TSHR blocking antibodies transfer across the placenta, which directly suppresses T3 and T4 production in the foetal thyroid (**Table 5**). Among these patient's neonatal hypothyroidism tends to be transient due to the clearance of the ATD and antibodies from the neonatal circulation; hence, they may not require treatment [78].

Central hypothyroidism arises from downregulation and delayed maturity of the foetal pituitary due to excessive production of thyroid hormones following foetal thyroid stimulation by maternal TRSAB. This tends to be transient in about 70% of the neonates; however, in 30% it may persist requiring lifelong treatment with levothyroxine [66, 79].

Pathological state	Targeted action of the medication	Pharmacological agents
Excessive adrenergic stimulation	Adrenergic blockage	Propranolol 0.25–0.75 mg/kg/dose 8hrly
Excessive adrenergic stimulation with cardiac failure	Reduction of preload, afterload, rate and rhythm control	Diuretics and digoxin
Excessive stimulation of the thyroid by TRabs	Blockage of thyroid hormone synthesis	PTU 5–10 mg/kg/day in 3 doses OR Carbimazole 0.5–1.5 mg/kg/day OR Methimazole 0.25–1 mg/kg/day in 2–3 divided doses
	Suppression of synthesis and release of thyroid hormones	Potassium 1–2 drops daily Lugol's solution 1 drop (8 mg) 8 hourly
Excessive levels of peripheral T3 and T4	Suppress peripheral conversion from T4 to T3 Compensation for thyroid hormone induced hyper-catabolism of endogenous glucocorticoids	Prednisone 2 mg/kg/day
Restlessness and irritability	Supportive care	Sedatives

Adapted from Ref. [68].

Table 4.
Treatment options for neonates with congenital hyperthyroidism.

Clinical condition	TSH	T4
Central congenital hypothyroidism	Low / normal or mildly elevated	Low
Primary congenital hypothyroidism	High	Low

Table 5.
Biochemical features of central and primary neonatal hypothyroidism.

8.4.1 Clinical features of neonates with congenital hypothyroidism

Most neonates with congenital hypothyroidism may be asymptomatic; however, symptoms include decreased motor activity, longer spells of sleeping, feeding difficulties, horse cry and prolonged jaundice. The physical examination may reveal enlarged fontanelles, macroglossia, hypotonia, rounded abdomen, umbilical hernia and myxoedema [80].

8.4.2 Management of neonates with congenital hypothyroidism

The recommended treatment should be L-T4 which should be initiated within the first 2 weeks of life at a dose of 10–15 mcg/kg/day according to severity of the disease and dose adjusted according to fT4 and TSH levels [81]. Close follow-up of 1–2 weeks is necessary till TSH levels are established then 1–3 months in the first year and then 2–4 months in the first 3 years. The target is to keep TSH levels within the normal limits according to age and fT4 levels in the upper half of the normal range [81].

9. Postpartum thyroiditis and depression

Postpartum thyroiditis is an autoimmune destructive inflammation of the thyroid gland that manifests within the first 12 months after delivery or miscarriage [82]. A fifth to one quarter of the patients present with the classic biphasic nature of thyrotoxicosis presenting within the first 1–4 months after delivery followed by hypothyroid state in the next 4–8 months. Another quarter present only with thyrotoxicosis, about 50% only with hypothyroid phases [41, 83]. About 80–85% revert to euthyroid state, the rest remaining hypothyroid [41, 83]. While postpartum thyroiditis is associated with a wide range of somatic and psychic symptoms, depression has been more associated with the hypothyroid phase, while anxiety and hyperactivity are more common in the thyrotoxicosis phase of this disease [83]. This may explain the conflicting results reported by different studies that sought to establish the relationship between postpartum thyroiditis and postpartum depression [84, 85] that may have had participants with differing phases of postpartum thyroiditis. Anticipation of the possible incidence of postpartum depression during the hypothyroid phase will help plan appropriate follow-up with consequent early diagnosis and management of women at risk of postpartum depression secondary to postpartum thyroiditis.

An increased incidence of thyroid autoimmunity has been reported following iodine supplementation among populations with mild-to-moderate iodine deficiency [7, 8]. The physiological diminution of cell-mediated immunity during pregnancy may mask the autoimmune thyroiditis, which may manifest as postpartum thyroiditis and with features of depression several months postpartum well past the puerperium period [4, 86]. Hence, it may be prudent to increase surveillance for postpartum thyroiditis and postpartum depression in populations undergoing iodine supplementation due to endemic mild-to-moderate iodine deficiency.

10. Conclusion

Although hyperthyroidism has limited impact on fecundity, if undiagnosed or not effectively controlled, it can greatly reduce fecundability for both fertile women and those on fertility treatment through early pregnancy losses and iatrogenic preterm delivery that may accompany maternal complications. The transient increase in hyperthyroidism secondary to iodine fortification is associated with higher incidence non-toxic and toxic thyroid nodules among women in later half of reproductive age and Graves' disease among younger women. This may not only increase the incidence of perinatal, congenital and behavioural complications associated with *in utero* exposure to ATD and TRabs, but also maternal mental and cardiovascular complications. This calls for more studies to further elucidate the epidemiology of hyperthyroidism and other thyroid disease especially in populations with recurrent waves of recurrent iodine deficiency or excess with concurrent iodine fortification as well as increased vigilance during prenatal and postnatal care. Poorly controlled hyperthyroidism in pregnancy is associated with maternal morbidity and mortality. Long follow-up of children born to mothers with hyperthyroidism is crucial as they may present with neurocognitive disorders.

Conflict of interest

The authors declare no conflict of interest.

Author details

Constance Nontsikelelo Gubu-Ntaba[1,2], Vulikhaya Mpumlwana[1,2], Nandipha Mizpa Sotobe-Mbana[1,3], Martha Mayer[1,3], Chukwuma Ogbonna Ekpebegh[1,4] and Charles Bitamazire Businge[1,2]*

1 Walter Sisulu University, Mthatha, South Africa

2 Department of Obstetrics and Gynaecology, Nelson Mandela Academic Hospital, Mthatha, Eastern Cape, South Africa

3 Department of Paediatrics, Nelson Mandela Academic Hospital, Mthatha, Eastern Cape, South Africa

4 Department of Internal Medicine, Nelson Mandela Academic Hospital, Mthatha, Eastern Cape, South Africa

*Address all correspondence to: cbusingae@gmail.com

References

[1] Yen PM. Physiological and molecular basis of thyroid hormone action. Physiological Reviews. 2001;**81**(3): 1097-1126

[2] Mintziori G, Kita M, Duntas L, Goulis DG. Consequences of hyperthyroidism in male and female fertility: Pathophysiology and current management. Journal of Endocrinological Investigation. 2016;**39**: 849-853

[3] De Leo S, Lee SY, Braverman LE. Hyperthyroidism. Lancet. 2016;**388** (10047):906-918

[4] Moleti M, Di Mauro M, Sturniolo G, Russo M, Vermiglio F. Hyperthyroidism in the pregnant woman: Maternal and fetal aspects. Journal of Clinical & Translational Endocrinology. 2019;**12** (16):100190. DOI: 10.1016/j.jcte.2019.100190

[5] Alves Junior JM, Bernardo WM, Ward LS, Villagelin D. Effect of hyperthyroidism control during pregnancy on maternal and Fetal outcome: A systematic review and meta-analysis. Frontiers in Endocrinology. 2022;**13**:800257. DOI: 10.3389/fendo.2022.800257

[6] Laurberg P, Cerqueira C, Ovesen L, Rasmussen LB, Perrild H, Andersen S, et al. Iodine intake as a determinant of thyroid disorders in populations. Best Practice & Research. Clinical Endocrinology & Metabolism. 2010;**24** (1):13-27

[7] Pedersen IB, Laurberg P, Knudsen N, Jorgensen T, Perrild H, Ovesen L, et al. Increase in incidence of hyperthyroidism predominantly occurs in young people after iodine fortification of salt in Denmark. The Journal of Clinical Endocrinology & Metabolism. 2006;**91** (10):3830-3834

[8] Sarfo-Kantanka O, Kyei I, Sarfo FS, Ansah EO. Thyroid disorders in Central Ghana: The influence of 20 years of iodization. Journal of Thyroid Research. 2017;**2017**:7843972. DOI: 10.1155/2017/7843972

[9] Wang C, Li Y, Teng D, Shi X, Ba J, Chen B, et al. Hyperthyroidism prevalence in China after universal salt iodization. Frontiers in Endocrinology. 2021;**12**:651534. DOI: 10.3389/fendo.2021.651534

[10] Laurberg P, Bülow Pedersen I, Knudsen N, Ovesen L, Andersen S. Environmental iodine intake affects the type of nonmalignant thyroid disease. Thyroid. 2001;**11**(5):457-469

[11] Petersen M, Knudsen N, Carlé A, Andersen S, Jørgensen T, Perrild H, et al. Thyrotoxicosis after iodine fortification: A 21-year Danish population-based study. Clinical Endocrinology. 2018;**89** (3):360-366

[12] Shan Z, Chen L, Lian X, Liu C, Shi B, Shi L, et al. Iodine status and prevalence of thyroid disorders after introduction of mandatory universal salt iodization for 16 years in China: A cross-sectional study in 10 cities. Thyroid. 2016;**26**(8):1125-1130

[13] Lazarus JH. Iodine status in Europe in 2014. European Thyroid Journal. 2014;**3**:3-6

[14] Zimmermann MB, Gizak M, Abbott K, Andersson M, Lazarus JH. Iodine deficiency in pregnant women in Europe. The Lancet Diabetes and Endocrinology. 2015;**3**:672-674

[15] Kung AW, Chau MT, Lao TT, Tam SC, Low LC. The effect of pregnancy on thyroid nodule formation. The Journal of Clinical Endocrinology and Metabolism. 2002;**87**:1010-1014

[16] Vitti P, Rago T, Tonacchera M, Pinchera A. Toxic multinodular goiter in the elderly. Journal of Endocrinological Investigation. 2002;**25**:16-18

[17] Taylor PN, Albrecht D, Scholz A, Gutierrez-Buey G, Lazarus JH, Dayan CM, et al. Global epidemiology of hyperthyroidism and hypothyroidism. Nature Reviews. Endocrinology. 2018;**14**(5):301-316

[18] Andersson M, Karumbunathan V, Zimmermann MB. Global iodine status in 2011 and trends over the past decade. The Journal of Nutrition. 2012;**142**(4): 744-750

[19] Volzke H, Erlund I, Hubalewska-Dydejczyk A, Ittermann T, Peeters RP, Rayman M, et al. How do we improve the impact of iodine deficiency disorders prevention in Europe and beyond? European Thyroid Journal. 2018;**7**(4): 193-200

[20] Howlett TA, Levy MJ. Endocrine disease. In: Kumar P, Clark M, editors. Kumar and Clark's Clinical Medicine. 7th ed. Vol. 18. Edinburgh. London. New York. Oxford. Philadelphia. St Louis. Sydney. Toronto: Saunders Elsevier; 2009. p. 9631027

[21] Nystrom HF, Jansson S, Berg G. Incidence rate and clinical features of hyperthyroidism in a long-term iodine sufficient area of Sweden (Gothenburg) 2003-2005. Clinical Endocrinology. 2013;**78**:768-776

[22] Marino M, Latrofa F, Menconi F, Chiovato L, Vitti P. Role of genetic and non-genetic factors in the etiology of Graves' disease. Journal of Endocrinological Investigation. 2015;**38**: 283-294

[23] Wiersinga WM. Smoking and thyroid. Clinical Endocrinology. 2013;**79**: 145-151

[24] Laurberg P, Nohr SB, Pedersen KM, et al. Thyroid disorders in mild iodine deficiency. Thyroid. 2000;**10**:951-963

[25] Laurberg P, Cerqueira C, Ovesen L, Rasmussen LB, Perrild H, Andersen S, et al. Iodine intake as a determinant of thyroid disorders in populations. Best Practice & Research. Clinical Endocrinology & Metabolism. 2010;**24**(1):13-27

[26] Zimmermann MB, Boelaert K. Iodine deficiency and thyroid disorders. The Lancet Diabetes and Endocrinology. 2015;**3**(4):286-295

[27] van Soestbergen MJ, van der Vijver JC, Graafland AD. Recurrence of hyperthyroidism in multinodular goiter after long-term drug therapy: A comparison with graves' disease. Journal of Endocrinological Investigation. 1992; **15**:797-800

[28] Yoshimura M, Hershman JM. Thyrotropic action of human chorionic gonadotropin. Thyroid. 1995;**5**(5):425-434. DOI: 10.1089/thy.1995.5.425

[29] Nguyen CT, Sasso EB, Barton L, Mestman JH. Graves' hyperthyroidism in pregnancy: A clinical review. Clinical Diabetes and Endocrinology. 2018;**4**:4. DOI: 10.1186/s40842-018-0054-7

[30] Wang JW, Liao XX, Li T. Thyroid autoimmunity in adverse fertility and pregnancy outcomes: Timing of assisted reproductive technology in AITD women: Journal of translational. Internal Medicine. 2021;**9**(2):76-83

[31] Davis LB, Lathi RB, Dahan MH. The effect of infertility medication on thyroid function in hypothyroid women who conceive. Thyroid. 2007;**17**:7737

[32] Pereira JVB, Lim T. Hyperthyroidism in gestational trophoblastic disease – A literature review. Thyroid Research. 2021;**14**(1): 1-7

[33] Karaca N, Akpak YM. Thyroid disorders and fertility: International. Journal of Research in Medical Sciences. 2015;**3**(6):1299-1304

[34] Krassas GE, Poppe K, Glinoer D. Thyroid function and human reproductive health. Endocrine Reviews. 2010;**31**(5):702-755

[35] Jeffereys A, Vanderpump M, Yasmin E. Thyroid dysfunction and reproductive health. The Obstetrician and Gynaecologist. 2015;**17**:39-45

[36] Unuane D, Velkeiers B. Impact of thyroid disease on fertility and assisted conception. Best Practice and Research Clinical Endocrinology and Metabolism. 2020;**34**:101378

[37] Zegers-Hochschild F, Adamson GD, de Mouzonj I, Mansour R, Nygraw K, Sullivan B, et al. ICMART/WHO revised glossary on ART terminology. Human Reproduction. 2009;**24**:2683-2687

[38] Sturgis SH, Lerman J, Stanbury JB. The menstrual pattern in thyroid disease. The Journal of Chinese Endocrinology & Metabolism. 1952;**12**:846-855

[39] Joshi JV, Bhandarkar SD, Chadha M, et al. Menstrual irregularities and lactation failure may precede thyroid dysfunction or goitre. Journal of Postgraduate Medicine. 1993;**39**: 137-141

[40] La Vignersa S, Vita R. Thyroid dysfunction and semen quality. International Journal of Immunopathology and Pharmacology. 2018;**32**:1-5

[41] Alexander EK, Pearce EN, Brent GA, Brown RS, Chen H, Dosiou C, et al. 2017 guidelines of the American Thyroid Association for the diagnosis and management of thyroid disease during pregnancy and the postpartum. Thyroid. 2017;**27**:315-389

[42] Gheorghiu ML, Bors RG, Gheorghisan-Galateanu AA, Pop AL, Cretoiu D, Varlas VN. Hyperthyroidism in pregnancy: The delicate balance between too much or too little antithyroid drug. Journal of Clinical Medicine. 2021;**10**(16):3742. DOI: 10.3390/jcm10163742

[43] Okosieme OE, Khan I, Taylor PN. Preconception management of thyroid dysfunction. Clinical Endocrinology. 2018;**89**(3):269-279. DOI: 10.1111/cen.13731

[44] Ross DS, Burch HB, Cooper DS, et al. 2016 American Thyroid Association guidelines for diagnosis and management of hyperthyroidism and other causes of thyrotoxicosis. Thyroid. 2016;**26**:1343-1421

[45] Wright H, Williams D. Thyrotoxicosis in pregnancy. Fetal and Maternal Medicine Review. 2013;**24**(2): 108-128

[46] Donna MN, Cootauco AC, Burrow G. Thyroid disease in pregnancy. Clinics in Perinatology. 2007;**34**:543-557

[47] Nisha Nathan MD, Shannon D, Sullivan. Thyroid disorders during pregnancy. Endocrinology and Metabolism Clinics of North America. 2014;**43**:573-597

[48] Cotzias C, Wong SJ, Taylor E, Seed P, Girling J. A study to establish gestation-specific reference intervals for thyroid function tests in normal singleton pregnancy. European Journal of Obstetrics, Gynecology, and Reproductive Biology. 2008;**137**(1): 61-66

[49] Cooper DS, Lauberg P. Hyperthyroidism in pregnancy. The Lancet Diabetes and Endocrinology. 2013;**3**:238-249

[50] Laurberg P, Vestergaard H, Nielsen S, Christensen SE, Seefeldt T, Helleberg K, et al. Sources of circulating 3,5,3′-triiodothyronine in hyperthyroidism estimated after blocking of type 1 and type 2 iodothyronine deiodinases. The Journal of Clinical Endocrinology and Metabolism. 2007;**92**(6):2149-2156

[51] Goldman AM, Mestman JH. Transient non-autoimmune hyperthyroidism of early pregnancy. Journal of Thyroid Research. 2011;**2011**: 142413

[52] Mestman JH. Hyperthyroidism in pregnancy. Current Opinion in Endocrinology, Diabetes, and Obesity. 2012;**19**:394-401

[53] Gargallo-Fernández M. Hyperthyroidism and pregnancy. Endocrinología y Nutrición. 2013;**60**: 535-543

[54] Negro R, Mestman JH. Thyroid disease in pregnancy. Best Practice & Research. Clinical Endocrinology & Metabolism. 2011;**25**(6):927-943

[55] Polak M, Luton D. Fetal thyroïdology. *Best practice & research*. Clinical Endocrinology & Metabolism. 2014;**28**(2):161-173. DOI: 10.1016/j.beem.2013.04.013

[56] Krassas G, Karras SN, Pontikides N. Thyroid diseases during pregnancy: A number of important issues. Hormones (Athens, Greece). 2015;**14**(1):59-69

[57] van Dijk MM, Smits IH, Fliers E, Bisschop PH. Maternal thyrotropin receptor antibody concentration and the risk of fetal and neonatal thyrotoxicosis: A systematic review. Thyroid. 2018;**28**(2):257-264

[58] Abeillon-du Payrat J, Chikh K, Bossard N, Bretones P, Gaucherand P, Claris O, et al. Predictive value of maternal second-generation thyroid-binding inhibitory immunoglobulin assay for neonatal autoimmune hyperthyroidism. European Journal of Endocrinology. 2014;**171**:451-460

[59] Andersen SL, Andersen S. Antithyroid drugs and birth defects. Thyroid Research. 2020;**13**:11. DOI: 10.1186/s13044-020-00085-8

[60] Kornacki J, Skrzypczak J. Fetal neck tumors - antenatal and intrapartum management. Ginekologia Polska. 2017; **88**(5):266-269

[61] Marx H, Amin P, Lazarus JH. Hyperthyroidism and pregnancy. BMJ. 2008;**336**(7645):663-667

[62] Huel C, Guibourdenche J, Vuillard E, Ouahba J, Piketty J, Oury JF, et al. Use of ultrasound to distinguish between fetal hyperthyroidism and hypothyroidism on discovery of a goiter. Ultrasound in Obstetrics & Gynecology. 2009;**33**:412-420

[63] Kurtoglu S, Ozdemir. Fetal neonatal hyperthyroidism: Diagnostic and therapeutic approachment. Turkish Archives of Pediatrics. 2017;**52**(1):1-9

[64] Hudzik B, Zubelewicz-Szkodzinska B. Antithyroid drugs during

breastfeeding. Clinical Endocrinology. 2016;**85**(6):827-830

[65] Segni M. Neonatal hyperthyroidism [updated 2019 Apr 15]. In: Feingold KR, Anawalt B, Boyce A, et al., editors. Endotext [Internet]. South Dartmouth (MA): MDText.com, Inc.; 2000 Available from: https://www.ncbi.nlm.nih.gov/books/NBK279019/

[66] Kurtoglu S, Ozdemir. Fetal neonatal hyperthyroidism: Diagnostic and therapeutic approachment. Turkish Archives of Pediatrics. 2017;**52**(1):1-9

[67] Törnhage CJ, Grankvist K. Acquired neonatal thyroid disease due to TSH receptor antibodies in breast milk. Journal of Pediatric Endocrinology and Metabolism. 2006;**19**(6):787-794

[68] van der Kaay DC, Wasserman JD, Palmert MR. Management of neonates born to mothers with Graves' disease. Pediatrics. 2016;**137**(4):e20151878

[69] Pyrżak B, Rumińska M, Witkowska-Sędek E, Kucharska A. Follow-up of thyroid function in children with neonatal hyperthyroidism. Frontiers in Endocrinology (Lausanne). 2022;**13**: 877119

[70] Papendieck P, Chiesa A, Prieto L, Gruñeiro-Papendieck L. Thyroid disorders of neonates born to mothers with Graves' disease. Journal of Pediatric Endocrinology & Metabolism. 2009;**22** (6):547-553

[71] Leger J. Management of fetal and neonatal Graves' disease. Hormone Research in Pædiatrics. 2017;**87**:1-6

[72] Polak M. Hyperthyroidism in early infancy: Pathogenesis, clinical features and diagnosis with a focus on neonatal hyperthyroidism. Thyroid. 1998;**8**: 1171-1177

[73] Ogilvy-Stuart AL. Neonatal thyrotoxicosis. NeoReviews. 2017;**18**(7): e422-e430

[74] Bucci I, Giuliani C, Napolitano G. Thyroid-stimulating hormone receptor antibodies in pregnancy: Clinical relevance. Frontiers in Endocrinology (Lausanne). 2017;**8**:137

[75] Neal PR, Jansen RD, Lemons JA, Mirkin LD, Schreiner RL. Unusual manifestations of neonatal hyperthyroidism. American Journal of Perinatology. 1985;**2**(03):231-235

[76] Samuels SL, Namoc SM, Bauer AJ. Neonatal thyrotoxicosis. Clinics in Perinatology. 2018;**45**(1):31-40

[77] Besancon A, Beltrand J, Le Gac I, Luton D, Polak M. Management of neonates born to women with Graves' disease: A cohort study. European Journal of Endocrinology. 2014;**170**(6): 855-862

[78] Kempers MJ, van Tijn DA, van Trotsenburg AS, de Vijlder JJ, Wiedijk BM, Vulsma T. Central congenital hypothyroidism due to gestational hyperthyroidism: Detection where prevention failed. The Journal of Clinical Endocrinology and Metabolism. 2003;**88** (12):5851-5857

[79] van Trotsenburg ASP. Management of neonates born to mothers with thyroid dysfunction, and points for attention during pregnancy. Best Practice & Research Clinical Endocrinology & Metabolism. 2020;**34**:101437

[80] Özon A, Tekin N, Şıklar Z, et al. Neonatal effects of thyroid diseases in pregnancy and approach to the infant with increased TSH: Turkish Neonatal and Pediatric Endocrinology and Diabetes Societies consensus report.

Turkish Archives of Pediatrics. 2018;**53** (Suppl 1):S209-S223

[81] van Trotsenburg P, Stoupa A, Leger J, Rohrer T, Peters C, et al. Congenital hypothyroidism: A 2020–2021 consensus guidelines update— An ENDO-European reference network initiative endorsed by the European Society for Pediatric Endocrinology and the European Society for Endocrinology. Thyroid. 2021;**31**(3):387-419

[82] Stagnaro-Green A. Approach to the patient with postpartum thyroiditis. The Journal of Clinical Endocrinology and Metabolism. 2012;**97**(2):334-342

[83] Argatska AB, Nonchev BI. Postpartum thyroiditis. Folia Med (Plovdiv). 2014;**56**(3):145-151

[84] Schmidt PMDS, Longoni A, Pinheiro RT, Assis AM. Postpartum depression in maternal thyroidal changes. Thyroid Research. 2022;**15**(1):6. DOI: 10.1186/s13044-022-00124-6

[85] Lucas A, Pizarro E, Granada ML, Salinas I, Sanmarti A. Postpartum thyroid dysfunction and postpartum depression: Are they two linked disorders? Clinical Endocrinology (Oxford). 2001;**55**:809-814

[86] De Leo S, Pearce EN. Autoimmune thyroid disease during pregnancy. The Lancet Diabetes and Endocrinology. 2018;**6**(7):575-586

Chapter 6

Thyrotoxic Hypokalemic Periodic Paralysis

Mustafa Cesur and Irmak Sayın Alan

Abstract

Thyrotoxic hypokalemic periodic paralysis (THPP) is a rare but life-threatening complication of hyperthyroidism characterized by recurrent episodes of muscle weakness due to intracellular potassium shifting in the presence of high levels of thyroid hormone. Attacks can be triggered by many factors. Its differential diagnosis from the other common causes of hypokalemic paralysis is necessary to maintain targeted therapy. Outcome was right away positive under potassium replacement therapy. Hyperthyroidism should be treated to prevent attacks.

Keywords: hypokalemia, periodic paralysis, thyrotoxicosis, pathophysiology of THPP, management of THPP

1. Introduction

Hypokalemia can be defined as a serum potassium level under 3.5 mEq/L. The symptoms of severe hypokalemia are nonspecific and mainly are related to muscular or cardiac functions and its effects on nerves. In severe and life-threatening hypokalemia (serum potassium of less than 2.5 mEq/L) generalized weakness and dangerous ventricular tachyarrhythmias may occur. Heart muscle can be affected by arrhythmias and may lead to heart failure [1, 2]. Acute decrease of serum potassium may be more arrhythmogenic than chronic hypokalemia [3].

Acute hypokalemic paralysis is a clinical syndrome presenting with low serum potassium levels and acute systemic weakness. The muscular weakness ranges from minor weakness to complete flaccid paralysis. This clinical syndrome is extremely rare. Fortunately, it is a treatable condition. Thyrotoxic hypokalemic periodic paralysis (THPP) is one of the reason of acute hypokalemic paralysis [4]. Approximately 32% of acute hypokalemic paralysis has found to be related to thyrotoxicosis [5].

The association between thyrotoxicosis and periodic paralysis was first described by Rosenfeld in 1902. THPP is a rare condition, which occurs in 2% of patients with thyrotoxicosis. THPP is mainly sporadic, but may be associated with certain HLA haplotypes [6]. There is no exact knowledge about genetic disposition of THPP. Genetic analysis identified heterozygous variants in candidate genes. But no single pathogenetic mutation has been identified. Several single-nucleotide polymorphisms in these genes have been associated with THPP. Determination of the complete

Triggering factors	
• Awakening in the middle of sleep	• Alcohol
• High carbohydrate intake	• Cold exposure
• High salt intake	• Drugs (diuretics, estrogen, laxatives, steroids and amphotericin B, etc.)
• Epinephrine	• Insulin
• Menstrual cycle	• Upper respiratory tract infections
• Radioactive iodine treatment	• Trauma
• Rest after strenuous exercise	• Surgery
• Emotional stress	
• Abuse of thyroid hormone	

Table 1.
Triggering factors of Thyrotoxic hypokalemic paralytic episodes.

genetic architecture in the future studies will be helpful to understand the pathophysiology of THPP [7, 8].

THPP is generally associated with intermittent episodes of muscle weakness and occasionally with severe paralysis. Paralytic attacks are mostly precipitated by strenuous exercise, high glucose intake, or hyperinsulinemia. THPP is a widespread complication of hyperthyroidism in males (85%) of Asian origin with a frequency of almost 2% [4, 9]. The case of THPP in the females is a rare occurrence. The reason for this is mysterious but proposes that androgens have a role in the pathogenesis of THPP. Cases with symptoms are generally between 20 and 40 years of age [10, 11]. Rarely it can be seen in children and adolescents [12] or elderly [13].

The best part of etiological agents for thyrotoxicosis may be related with THPP. The major agent was reported to be Graves' disease [12, 13]. Silent thyroiditis and subacute thyroiditis are the rest etiologies [4]. THPP related with Coronavirus disease 2019 (Covid-19) infection reported in some data. Higher incidence of hyperthyroidism was reported in patients with Covid-19 infection, probably related to immune response to the infection. Thyroid function was shown to be improved when the infection was resolved [14, 15].

Various circumstances, including TSH-secreting pituitary adenoma [16], using high doses of thyroxine [17, 18], and iodine-related thyrotoxicosis with inattentive use of iodine or with drugs containing iodine (e.g., iodinate contrast agents or amiodarone) [19–21] have also been involved.

One of the Turkish cases occurred as the first manifestation of interferon-alpha-induced Graves' disease [22] while another occurred after radioactive iodine therapy, which led to the consideration of radiation thyroiditis [23]. There are many triggering factors [4, 24, 25]. The triggering factors of thyrotoxic hypokalemic paralytic episodes are given in **Table 1**.

2. The pathophysiology of THPP

The pathophysiology of THPP is poorly understood. In THPP, flaccid paralysis occurs with comparatively minor alterings in the serum potassium level. Hypokalemia is the characteristic evidence with elevated thyroid hormones. It is generated with a quick shift in K from the extracellular space to the intracellular department, particularly into the muscles. Increased adrenergic responses and elevated circulating levels of insulin and thyroid hormones raise Na^+/K^+-ATPase activity. Additionally, thyroid hormones rise the sensitivity of beta-receptors, so catecholamine-mediated cellular K uptake is raised [26, 27]. These suggestions may explain why insulin and epinephrine stimulate paralytic attacks. Carbohydrate-rich meals increase insulin release, and stress-related factors (e.g., emotional stress, cold, trauma, and infection) increase epinephrine delivery. Exercise also delivers K from the skeletal muscles, while rest encourages flow of K, so paralytic attacks may be seen during rest after strenuous exercise [28].

The robust preference for THPP to occur in males brings forward that androgens may take part to pathogenesis of THPP. Androgens have been reported to enhance the expression and activity of the Na^+/K^+-ATPase and hence related with TPP attacks [29]. Potassium channel Kir2.6 gene mutations have been established to take a role in THPP. Kir2.6 is mainly expressed in skeletal muscle and is transcriptionally arranged by thyroid hormone. Mutation of the gene coding this channel has been established in THPP cases and is related with high prevalence of paralytic attacks in those patients [30].

3. Differential diagnosis

In an acute attack, THPP must be distinguished from other causes of acute hypokalemic paralysis. Hypokalemic paralysis symbolizes a heterogeneous category of disorders, which cause an ultimate mutual pathway existing as acute weakness and hypokalemia. Hypokalemic paralysis can be divided into two main groups. The first group contains the patients with hypokalemic periodic paralysis, which is related to

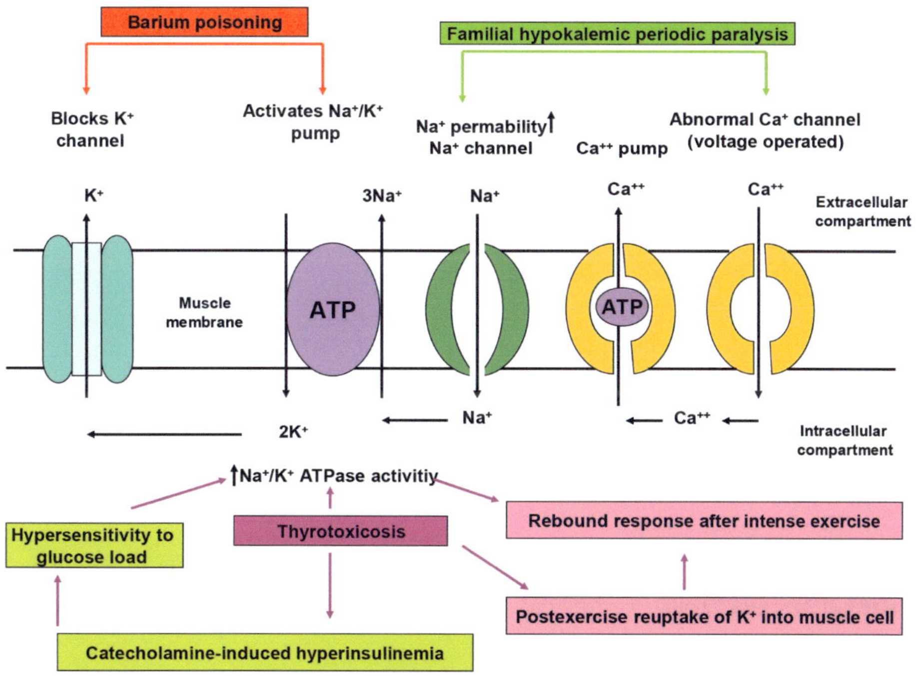

Figure 1.
Pathogenesis of hypokalaemic paralysis in transcellular distribution of potassium without depletion.

Transcellular distribution of potassium (no depletion)	Actual potassium depletion	
	Renal loss	Extra-renal loss
• Familial periodic paralysis	• Distal RTA	• Celiac disease
• Thyrotoxic periodic paralysis	• Sjögren's syndrome	• Tropical sprue
• Barium poisoning	• Medullary sponge kidney	• Severe diarrhea
	• Chronic toluene exposure	• Short bowel syndrome
	• Fanconi's syndrome	
	• Primary aldosteronism	

Table 2.
Differential diagnosis of hypokalemic paralysis.

an acute exchange of potassium into the cells (**Figure 1**). The second group contains the patients presenting with hypokalemic paralysis, which is related to potassium depletion. Diagnosis among paralytic attacks is hard as the patient may have normal force and potassium levels. Electromyography shows unusualness in a few patients but is frequently normal, particularly among episodes when no clinically detectable weakness is present. Hypokalemic paralysis happens in different situations, and the diagnosis may require a broad research for the underlying etiology since the treatment changes according to the reason [31].

The diagnosis of THPP is made based on clinical presentation and exclusion of disorders associated with low potassium (**Table 2**).

4. Clinical features

THPP attacks mostly occur in the late night or early morning and last from a few hours up to several days. Prodromal symptoms such as aches, cramps, and stiffness can be seen [32]. Generally, the proximal muscles are more seriously affected than the distal muscles. The acute episode at first involves the lower limbs, followed by girdle muscles and thereafter upper limb. Atypical findings such as asymmetric paralysis are uncommon. Presentations alter widely from mild, transient, self-limited motor dysfunction to total flaccid paralysis, with recovery occurring first in those muscles affected last. Bladder, bowel, and sensory functions are generally not affected and mental skills are never damaged [10]. Paralysis of respiratory, bulbar, and ocular muscles has been rarely reported in severe attacks of THPP. Respiratory muscle involvement, even though rare, generally can be fatal [33]. Deep tendon reflexes are prominently reduced or absent. Moriyama et al. reported that sudden deafness in a man with THPP, circulatory failure, and electrolyte instability in the right inner ear was accepted to have caused the deafness [34]. Patients completely recover between the attacks [26].

5. Laboratory features

Hypokalemia is the main laboratory finding in THPP. However, normokalemic THPP cases have also been reported [35, 36]. Normokalemia may lead to overlooked diagnosis [36]. The level of hypokalemia is important [31]. Serum potassium level may be one of the markers of survey of the disease for its reasoning of fatal and life-threatening ventricular arrhythmias [37, 38]. Hypomagnesemia and hypophosphatemia have been reported to be common in THPP. These laboratory results may aid differentiate THPP from familial hypokalemic periodic paralysis [39]. Elevated serum T3 and T4, low serum TSH levels, and thyroid uptake scan showing symmetric diffuse uptake are component of the diagnostic assessment. Patients with elevated T3 and normal T4 levels have been reported, particularly in patients who have Graves' disease or an adenoma who usually have T3 thyrotoxicosis [40]. Serum creatine phosphokinase (CPK) was found to be high [39, 41]. Rhabdomyolysis may be seen in severe THPP [42]. In addition to hypokalemia [43] and hypophosphataemia [44], hyperthyroidism alone may cause rhabdomyolysis [45]. ECG alterations in THPP vary from nondiagnostic to those demonstrating typical features of hypokalemia [46]. ECG alterations related with hypokalemia and/or other ECG abnormalities may be seen. ECG findings may help in early diagnosis of THPP [47, 48]. Sinus tachycardia, ventricular tachycardia, ventricular fibrillation, high QRS voltage, first-degree AV block, atrial flutter, and atrial fibrillation are significant signs proposing THPP in patients who present with paralysis and hypokalemia [48–50]. An artificial-intelligence-assisted-ECG system trustworthy recognizes hypokalemia in patients with paralysis, and combining with routine blood tests makes precious judgment assistance for the early diagnosis of THPP [51].

6. Management

Patients with acute paralysis must be hospitalized in a monitored condition for cardiac arrhythmias. Acute management of THPP contains potassium chloride replacement, cautious observation, and close monitoring of serum potassium levels. Potassium replacement can be done in two ways: oral or intravenous. A recommended protocol is 30 mEq of oral potassium every 2 hours until recovery begins, with a maximum dose of 90 mEq in 24 hours. Intravenous supplementation is the major choice if the patient shows signs of cardiac dysrhythmia, respiratory distress or is unable to take oral medications. The dosage of potassium varies between patients and can be standardized according to renal clearance and cardiovascular condition. Potassium replacement should not exceed 90 mEq/24 h because of the possibility of rebound hyperkalemia. Rebound hyperkalemia appears to be an important trouble in THPP, taking place in approximately 40–59% of treated attacks [4, 10, 52, 53]. In contrast to familial periodic paralysis, regular oral potassium supplementation is ineffective for prevention of the attacks in THPP [53]. Imminent monitoring of serum potassium levels throughout the acute attack is necessary. Continual cardiac monitoring is suggested for all patients throughout medical management and observation. A cardiology consultation should be provided for serious arrhythmias/ECG changes. Correction of hypomagnesemia, if present, is additionally suggested.

The best way to prevent and to permanently treat the periodic paralysis is to treat the thyrotoxicosis permanently. THPP does not disappear completely unless patients become euthyroid. Thus, the management of hyperthyroidism is the mainstay of therapy. Permanent treatment is so important and could be done by antithyroid drugs, radioiodine therapy, or surgery [27]. During treatment of hyperthyroidism, precipitating factors should be avoided. While antithyroid drugs may be used to induce remission, the performance of this therapy is changeable and relapses are frequent. By the end of the acute attack, radioiodine therapy or thyroid surgery is preferable to permanently end the thyrotoxicosis. For high recurrence rates of long-term treatment with antithyroid drugs, early permanent therapy, especially with radioactive iodine, is recommended because surgical stress may further induce paralysis. However, surgical therapy with close monitoring can be performed if necessary [4]. Chemical ablation has mainly shown benefit in elderly individuals, pregnant, cardiac and pediatric patients [54]. Non-selective beta-blockers (e.g., propranolol) have been shown to significantly improve thyrotoxic symptoms and maintain relief of paralytic attacks by blocking catecholamines' effect on ion channels [55]. Selective β-blockers do not act on skeletal muscle, which makes them less beneficial in the treatment of THPP [27]. In spite of likely benefits, beta-blockers (principally non-selective agents) are known to have a mild deleterious effect other metabolic parameters [56].

The effects of glucocorticoids in the management of hyperthyroidism have been evaluated in many different studies. Even though glucocorticoids have been used to treat hyperthyroidism, they may further cause harmful effects, including the development of THPP.

Glucocorticoids may induce hypokalemia by increasing the Na^+/K^+-ATPase level in skeletal muscle and also by creating hyperinsulinemia. In addition, glucocorticoids can also release muscle weakness by stimulating myopathy and renal potassium waste owing to its mineralocorticoid effects [11]. Consequently, glucocorticoids can trigger these attacks. This is an infrequent complication of thyrotoxicosis. But for physicians, it is important to be aware of the risk of provoking thyrotoxic paralysis when using high-dose glucocorticoids in the thyrotoxic phase [57]. Lastly, acetazolamide may worsen the attacks in THPP and should be avoided [52].

In conclusion, THPP is rare but life-threatening complication of thyrotoxicosis. It needs early diagnosis and immediate treatment of hypokalemia, then permanent therapy of thyrotoxicosis.

Author details

Mustafa Cesur[1]* and Irmak Sayın Alan[2]

1 Endocrinology and Metabolic Disease Department, Ankara Guven Hospital, Ankara, Türkiye

2 Internal Medicine Department, Ankara Guven Hospital, Ankara, Türkiye

*Address all correspondence to: drcesur@yahoo.com

References

[1] Kardalas E, Paschou SA, Anagnostis P, Muscogiuri G, Siasos G, Vryonidou A. Hypokalemia: a clinical update. Endocrine Connections. 2018;7(4):R135-R146. DOI: 10.1530/EC-18-0109

[2] Skogestad J, Aronsen JM. Hypokalemia-induced arrhythmias and heart failure: New ınsights and ımplications for therapy. Frontiers in Physiology. 2018;**9**:1500. DOI: 10.3389/fphys.2018.01500

[3] Shapiro JI, Banerjee A, Reiss OK, Elkins N. Acute and chronic hypokalemia sensitize the isolated heart to hypoxic injury. The American Journal of Physiology. 1998;**274**(5):H1598-H1604. DOI: 10.1152/ajpheart.1998.274.5.H1598

[4] Cesur M, Bayram F, Temel MA, Ozkaya M, Kocer A, Ertorer ME, et al. Thyrotoxic hypokalaemic periodic paralysis in a Turkish population: Three new case reports and analysis of the case series. Clinical Endocrinology. 2008;**68**(1):143-152. DOI: 10.1111/j.1365-2265.2007.03014.x

[5] Veltri KT, Mason C. Mcdication-induced hypokalemia. Pharmacy and Therapeutics. 2015;**40**(3):185-190

[6] Tamai H, Tanaka K, Komaki G, Matsubayashi S, Hirota Y, Mori K, et al. HLA and thyrotoxic periodic paralysis in Japanese patients. The Journal of Clinical Endocrinology and Metabolism. 1987;**64**(5):1075-1078. DOI: 10.1210/jcem-64-5-1075

[7] Rasheed E, Seheult J, Gibney J, Boran G. Does thyrotoxic periodic paralysis have a genetic predisposition? A case report. Annals of Clinical Biochemistry. 2018;**55**(6):713-716. DOI: 10.1177/0004563218785395

[8] Zhao SX, Liu W, Liang J, Gao GQ, Zhang XM, Yao Y, et al. China consortium for the genetics of autoimmune thyroid disease. Assessment of molecular subtypes in Thyrotoxic periodic paralysis and graves disease among Chinese Han adults: A population-based genome-wide association study. JAMA Network Open. 2019;**2**(5):e193348. DOI: 10.1001/jamanetworkopen.2019.3348

[9] Ahlawat SK, Sachdev A. Hypokalaemic paralysis. Postgraduate Medical Journal. 1999;**75**(882):193-197. DOI: 10.1136/pgmj.75.882.193

[10] Tinker TD, Vannatta JB. Thyrotoxic hypokalemic periodic paralysis: Report of four cases and review of the literature (1). The Journal of the Oklahoma State Medical Association. 1987;**80**(1):11-15

[11] El-Hennawy AS, Nesa M, Mahmood AK. Thyrotoxic hypokalemic periodic paralysis triggered by high carbohydrate diet. American Journal of Therapeutics. 2007;**14**(5):499-501. DOI: 10.1097/MJT.0b013e31814daf53

[12] Roh JG, Park KJ, Lee HS, Hwang JS. Thyrotoxic hypokalemic periodic paralysis due to Graves' disease in 2 adolescents. Annals of Pediatric Endocrinology & Metabolism. 2019;**24**(2):133-136. DOI: 10.6065/apem.2019.24.2.133

[13] Bilha S, Mitu O, Teodoriu L, Haba C, Preda C. Thyrotoxic periodic paralysis-a misleading challenge in the emergency department. Diagnostics (Basel). 2020;**10**(5):316. DOI: 10.3390/diagnostics10050316

[14] Khoo B, Tan T, Clarke SA, Mills EG, Patel B, Modi M, et al. Thyroid function

before, during, and after COVID-19. The Journal of Clinical Endocrinology and Metabolism. 2021;**106**(2):e803-e811. DOI: 10.1210/clinem/dgaa830

[15] Fitriani F, Susanti VY, Ikhsan MR. COVID-19 infection-related Thyrotoxic hypokalemic periodic paralysis. Case Reports in Endocrinology. 2022;**2022**:1382270. DOI: 10.1155/2022/1382270

[16] Alings AM, Fliers E, de Herder WW, Hofland LJ, Sluiter HE, Links TP, et al. A thyrotropin-secreting pituitary adenoma as a cause of thyrotoxic periodic paralysis. Journal of Endocrinological Investigation. 1998;**21**(10):703-706. DOI: 10.1007/BF03350802

[17] Chen YC, Fang JT, Chang CT, Chou HH. Thyrotoxic periodic paralysis in a patient abusing thyroxine for weight reduction. Renal Failure. 2001;**23**(1):139-142. DOI: 10.1081/jdi-100001294

[18] Patel AJ, Tejera S, Klek SP, Rothberger GD. Thyrotoxic peiıodic paralysis in a competitive bodybuilder with thyrotoxicosis factitia. AACE Clinical Case Reports. 2020;**6**(5):e252-e256. DOI: 10.4158/ACCR-2020-0154

[19] Tran HA. Inadvertent iodine excess causing thyrotoxic hypokalemic periodic paralysis. Archives of Internal Medicine. 2005;**165**(21):2536. DOI: 10.1001/archinte.165.21.2536-a

[20] Kane MP, Busch RS. Drug-induced thyrotoxic periodic paralysis. The Annals of Pharmacotherapy. 2006;**40**(4): 778-781. DOI: 10.1345/aph.1G543

[21] Laroia ST, Zaw KM, Ganti AK, Newman W, Akinwande AO. Amiodarone-induced thyrotoxicosis presenting as hypokalemic periodic paralysis. Southern Medical Journal. 2002;**95**(11):1326-1328

[22] Cesur M, Gursoy A, Avcioglu U, Erdogan MF, Corapcioglu D, Kamel N. Thyrotoxic hypokalemic periodic paralysis as the first manifestation of interferon-alpha-induced graves disease. Journal of Clinical Gastroenterology. 2006;**40**(9):864-865. DOI: 10.1097/01.mcg.0000212660.59021.a3

[23] Akar S, Comlekci A, Birlik M, Onen F, Sari I, Gurler O, et al. Thyrotoxic periodic paralysis in a Turkish male; the recurrence of the attack after radioiodine treatment. Endocrine Journal. 2005;**52**(1):149-151. DOI: 10.1507/endocrj.52.149

[24] Lin SH. Thyrotoxic periodic paralysis. Mayo Clinic Proceedings. 2005;**80**(1):99-105. DOI: 10.1016/S0025-6196(11)62965-0

[25] Mellgren G, Bleskestad IH, Aanderud S, Bindoff L. Thyrotoxicosis and paraparesis in a young woman: Case report and review of the literature. Thyroid. 2002;**12**(1):77-80. DOI: 10.1089/105072502753452002

[26] Cesur M, Ilgin SD, Baskal N, Gullu S. Hypokalemic paralysis is not just a hypokalemic paralysis. European Journal of Emergency Medicine. 2008;**15**(3):150-153. DOI: 10.1097/MEJ.0b013e3282bf6ee3

[27] Kung AW. Clinical review: Thyrotoxic periodic paralysis: A diagnostic challenge. The Journal of Clinical Endocrinology and Metabolism. 2006;**91**(7):2490-2495. DOI: 10.1210/jc.2006-0356

[28] Ober KP. Thyrotoxic periodic paralysis in the United States. Report of 7 cases and review of the literature. Medicine (Baltimore). 1992;**71**(3):109-120. DOI:10.1097/00005792-199205000-00001

[29] Biering H, Bauditz J, Pirlich M, et al. Manifestation of thyrotoxic periodic

paralysis in two patients with adrenal adenomas and hyperandrogenaemia. Hormone Research. 2003;**59**(6):301-304

[30] Ryan DP, da Silva MR, Soong TW, Fontaine B, Donaldson MR, Kung AW, et al. Mutations in potassium channel Kir2.6 cause susceptibility to thyrotoxic hypokalemic periodic paralysis. Cell. 2010;**140**(1):88-98. DOI: 10.1016/j.cell.2009.12.024

[31] Stedwell RE, Allen KM, Binder LS. Hypokalemic paralyses: A review of the etiologies, pathophysiology, presentation, and therapy. The American Journal of Emergency Medicine. 1992;**10**(2):143-148. DOI: 10.1016/0735-6757(92)90048-3

[32] Sanyal D, Bhattacharjee S. Thyrotoxic hypokalemic periodic paralysis as the presenting symptom of silent thyroiditis. Annals of Indian Academy of Neurology. 2013;**16**(2):218-220. DOI: 10.4103/0972-2327.112471

[33] Liu YC, Tsai WS, Chau T, Lin SH. Acute hypercapnic respiratory failure due to thyrotoxic periodic paralysis. The American Journal of the Medical Sciences. 2004;**327**(5):264-267. DOI:10.1097/00000441-200405000-00025

[34] Moriyama K, Nozaki M, Kudo J, Takita A, Tatewaki E, Yasuda K. Sudden deafness in a man with thyrotoxic hypokalemic periodic paralysis. Japanese Journal of Medicine. 1988;**27**(3):329-332. DOI: 10.2169/internalmedicine1962.27.329

[35] González-Treviño O, Rosas-Guzmán J. Normokalemic thyrotoxic periodic paralysis: A new therapeutic strategy. Thyroid. 1999;**9**(1):61-63. DOI: 10.1089/thy.1999.9.61

[36] Wu CC, Chau T, Chang CJ, Lin SH. An unrecognized cause of paralysis in ED: Thyrotoxic normokalemic periodic paralysis. The American Journal of Emergency Medicine. 2003;**21**(1):71-73. DOI: 10.1053/ajem.2003.50005

[37] Randall BB. Fatal hypokalemic thyrotoxic periodic paralysis presenting as the sudden, unexplained death of a Cambodian refugee. The American Journal of Forensic Medicine and Pathology. 1992;**13**(3):204-206. DOI: 10.1097/00000433-199209000-00006

[38] Loh KC, Pinheiro L, Ng KS. Thyrotoxic periodic paralysis complicated by near-fatal ventricular arrhythmias. Singapore Medical Journal. 2005;**46**(2):88-88

[39] Manoukian MA, Foote JA, Crapo LM. Clinical and metabolic features of thyrotoxic periodic paralysis in 24 episodes. Archives of Internal Medicine. 1999;**159**(6):601-606. DOI: 10.1001/archinte.159.6.601

[40] Griggs RC, Bender AN, Tawil R. A puzzling case of periodic paralysis. Muscle & Nerve. 1996;**19**(3):362-364. DOI: 10.1002/(SICI)1097-4598(199603)19:3<362::AID-MUS13>3.0.CO;2-U

[41] Sabau I, Canonica A. Hypokalaemic periodic paralysis associated with controlled thyrotoxicosis. Schweizerische Medizinische Wochenschrift. 2000;**130**(44):1689-1691

[42] Kilpatrick RE, Seiler-Smith S, Levine SN. Thyrotoxic hypokalemic periodic paralysis: Report of four cases in black American males. Thyroid. 1994;**4**(4):441-445. DOI: 10.1089/thy.1994.4.441

[43] Singhal PC, Abramovici M, Venkatesan J, Mattana J. Hypokalemia and rhabdomyolysis. Mineral and Electrolyte Metabolism. 1991;**17**(5):335-339

[44] Amanzadeh J, Reilly RF Jr. Hypophosphatemia: An evidence-based approach to its clinical consequences and management. Nature Clinical Practice. Nephrology. 2006;**2**(3):136-148. DOI: 10.1038/ncpneph0124

[45] Lichtstein DM, Arteaga RB. Rhabdomyolysis associated with hyperthyroidism. The American Journal of the Medical Sciences. 2006;**332**(2):103-105. DOI: 10.1097/00000441-200608000-00012

[46] Ee B, Cheah JS. Electrocardiographic changes in thyrotoxic periodic paralysis. Journal of Electrocardiology. 1979;**12**(3):263-279. DOI: 10.1016/s0022-0736(79)80059-x

[47] Ngo A, Lim SH, Charles RA, Goh SH. Electrocardiographical case. Young man with generalised myalgia. Singapore Medical Journal. 2005;**46**(1):38-40

[48] Hsu YJ, Lin YF, Chau T, Liou JT, Kuo SW, Lin SH. Electrocardiographic manifestations in patients with thyrotoxic periodic paralysis. The American Journal of the Medical Sciences. 2003;**326**(3):128-132. DOI: 10.1097/00000441-200309000-00004

[49] Tsai IH, Su YJ. Thyrotoxic periodic paralysis with ventricular tachycardia. Journal of Electrocardiology. 2019;**54**:93-95. DOI: 10.1016/j.jelectrocard.2019.04.001 Epub 2019 Apr 4

[50] Sanchez-Nadales A, Celis-Barreto V, Diaz-Sierra A, Sanchez-Nadales A, Lewis A, Sleiman J. When cardiology meets endocrinology: Sustained atrial flutter associated with thyrotoxic periodic paralysis. Oxford Medical Case Reports. 2022;**2022**(3):omac020. DOI: 10.1093/omcr/omac020

[51] Lin C, Lin CS, Lee DJ, Lee CC, Chen SJ, Tsai SH, et al. Artificial intelligence-assisted electrocardiography for early diagnosis of Thyrotoxic periodic paralysis. Journal of the Endocrine Society. 2021;**5**(9):bvab120. DOI: 10.1210/jendso/bvab120

[52] Lu KC, Hsu YJ, Chiu JS, Hsu YD, Lin SH. Effects of potassium supplementation on the recovery of thyrotoxic periodic paralysis. The American Journal of Emergency Medicine. 2004;**22**(7):544-547. DOI: 10.1016/j.ajem.2004.09.016

[53] Cope TE, Samaraweera AP, Burn DJ. Thyrotoxic periodic paralysis: Correct hypokalemia with caution. The Journal of Emergency Medicine. 2013;**45**(3):338-340. DOI: 10.1016/j.jemermed.2012.11.107

[54] Baskin HJ, Cobin RH, Duick DS, Gharib H, Guttler RB, Kaplan MM, et al. American Association of Clinical Endocrinologists medical guidelines for clinical practice for the evaluation and treatment of hyperthyroidism and hypothyroidism. Endocrine Practice. 2002;**8**(6):457-469. DOI: 10.4158/1934-2403-8.6.457

[55] Shayne P, Hart A. Thyrotoxic periodic paralysis terminated with intravenous propranolol. Annals of Emergency Medicine. 1994;**24**(4):736-740. DOI: 10.1016/s0196-0644(94)70286-1

[56] Cooper-DeHoff RM, Pacanowski MA, Pepine CJ. Cardiovascular therapies and associated glucose homeostasis: Implications across the dysglycemia continuum. Journal of the American College of Cardiology. 2009;**53**(5

Suppl):S28-S34. DOI: 10.1016/j.jacc.2008.10.037

[57] Tigas S, Papachilleos P, Ligkros N, Andrikoula M, Tsatsoulis A. Hypokalemic paralysis following administration of intravenous methylprednisolone in a patient with Graves' thyrotoxicosis and ophthalmopathy. Hormones (Athens, Greece). 2011;**10**(4):313-316. DOI: 10.14310/horm.2002.1323

Chapter 7

Association of Micronutrients and Prevalence of Antibodies in Hyperthyroidism

Hari Krishnan Krishnamurthy, Swarnkumar Reddy, Vasanth Jayaraman, Karthik Krishna, Karenah E. Rajasekaran, Tianhao Wang, Kang Bei and John J. Rajasekaran

Abstract

Thyroid hormones play a pivotal role in the overall physiological and developmental function of the human body. Alterations in thyroid hormones drastically affect regular metabolic processes as well as physical well-being. Thyroid alterations directly influence the functioning of all major body systems including cardiovascular, neurological, gastrointestinal, etc. The thyroid hormonal imbalance is primarily classified into two major conditions: hyperthyroidism and hypothyroidism. The present chapter details the pathology of thyroid imbalance in the context of human reproductive health, autoimmunity, and micronutrient imbalance. Some novel micronutrient associations independent of iodine deficiencies are discussed. Additionally, the early predictive capability of the anti-TPO antibody as well as other autoimmune correlations are discussed. Given its role in reproductive health, the associations of various sex hormones with thyroid function were also explored.

Keywords: hyperthyroidism, micronutrients, Graves' disease, iodine, hormones, antibodies

1. Introduction

Thyroid disorders are the most common type of endocrine dysfunction worldwide, with an estimated prevalence of 5–6% in the US population. Thyroid disorders can be highly differentiated from other endocrine diseases in terms of diagnosis, accessibility of treatment methods, etc. [1]. Early diagnosis and treatment of thyroid diseases remain a cornerstone of management. It's well known that thyroid hormones play crucial roles in regulating various metabolic processes. Thyroid hormone synthesis is a sensitive and feedback loop-dependent system controlled by the hypothalamus-pituitary-thyroid (HPT) axis. The regular functioning of the thyroid gland is a delicate balance among the hypothalamus, pituitary gland, and the thyroid gland [2]. The feedback loop slows down the production of thyrotropin-releasing hormone (TRH) in the hypothalamus which in turn slows down the production of thyroid-stimulating hormone and down-regulates thyroid hormone when excess is synthesized [3], the reverse happens when the thyroid hormones are low. Any biochemical alterations in this feedback loop results in under-function or over-function of the thyroid gland resulting in catastrophic health consequences [4, 5]. Thyroid disease results from a broad spectrum of pathologies including autoimmune disorders, infectious diseases, organ damage, pharmaceutical compounds, nutritional deficiencies, and environmental factors.

Deficiency of nutrients, in particular micronutrients, results in various non-specific physiological effects including metabolic disorders, suppressed immune responses, and altered endocrine functioning—including that of the thyroid gland. Micronutrients play a key role in enzyme synthesis, immune function, and regulating cellular homeostasis [6, 7]. Optimum levels of iodine intake have long been associated with thyroid health, it is, however, important to consider the optimal supply of other micronutrients that aid in thyroid function as well.

Recent studies have demonstrated the early diagnosis of autoimmune thyroid diseases could reduce the severity of the consequent thyroid disease and reduce its effect on the resulting comorbid conditions. Autoimmune thyroid disease is the most common thyroid disorder affecting the reproductive system in both males and females resulting in infertility. The current chapter details the most important causes of thyroid dysfunction and also discusses recent advances in thyroid research covering various aspects. The application of anti-TPO as an early predictor of various thyroid disorders and the effect of thyroid alteration on human reproductive health is also discussed [8, 9].

2. The pathology of hyperthyroidism

Hyperthyroidism is characterized by exceedingly high secretions of free thyroxine (T4), triiodothyronine, or both. The elevated levels of thyroid hormone in tissues result in systemic clinical manifestations such as weight loss, palpitations, and heat intolerance that result in thyrotoxicosis [10]. Graves' disease, toxic multinodular goiters, and toxic adenomas are the most common causes of hyperthyroidism resulting from mutations in genes that regulate the TSH receptor causing familial or non-autoimmune hyperthyroidism (FNAH) [11]. In FNAH the disease-causing mutations are inherited in an autosomal dominant manner and distinguished by a positive history of inherited non-autoimmune hyperthyroidism exhibiting variable onset symptoms. With FNAH, patients are clinically presented with goiter with no signs of autoimmune responses. Iodine-induced hyperthyroidism is one of the major nutritional causes of hyperthyroidism. Others include germ cell tumors, thyroid cancer, trophoblastic, struma ovarii, TSH-producing pituitary tumors, and medications such as lithium or pregnancy. Hyperthyroidism resulting from these reasons is generally self-limited for a period of time and does not require any medications [12, 13].

3. Etiology and epidemiology

Hyperthyroidism is a clinical state resulting from the disproportionate secretion of thyroid hormones. The most common causes include Graves' disease and toxic nodular goiter and other less common causes include factitious thyroiditis, iodine-induced hyperthyroidism, subacute thyroiditis, and postpartum thyroiditis [14]. Graves' disease is the most common cause of hyperthyroidism in the United States and other western countries. The etiology of Graves' disease remains multifactorial, as it arises by the loss of immunotolerance resulting in the development of autoimmune responses this induces the thyroid follicular cells by binding to TSH receptors, Graves' disease is the most common cause of hyperthyroidism in the young population. Deficiency of vitamin D and selenium, thyroid damage, immunomodulating drugs, beta-blockers, and infections also account for the development of Graves' disease [15]. Toxic multinodular goiter was found to be the most common cause of hyperthyroidism in the older population [16]. The use of excessive pharmaceutical thyroid hormones or inappropriate intake of external hormones results in factitious thyroiditis. Due to a well-received side effect of weight loss, thyroxine has the potential for abuse, and any history of a hyperthyroid patient should include a medication list and an assessment of possible misuse (whether intentional or unintentional). Struma ovarii, metastatic follicular thyroid cancer, and TSH-secreting pituitary adenoma are the other less common causes of hyperthyroidism [16].

The global epidemiology of hyperthyroidism can be defined in correspondence to the population in iodine-deficient regions and iodine-sufficient regions. In Europe, the dietary intake of iodine is the major cause of hyperthyroidism, whereas in a few cases autoimmune disease results in hyperthyroidism. In the US, Grave's disease is the most common factor of hypothyroidism in the younger population, whereas toxic nodular goiter is more common among the older. The overall prevalence of hyperthyroidism is 0.8% and 1.3% in Europe and the USA respectively. The prevalence of overt hyperthyroidism rates 0.1 per 1000 men and 0.4 per 1000 women in Europe, whereas overt hyperthyroidism accounts for 0.5% of the total US population.

4. Forms of thyroid diseases

4.1 Graves' disease

Graves' disease is seen as the prime cause of hyperthyroidism and accounts for more than 70% of all hyperthyroid cases. Annually over 2% of women and 0.2% of men were reported with Graves' disease globally [17]. Graves' disease was found to be much more frequent in females, particularly during childhood, and more prevalent during puberty. The pathology of Graves' disease remains unclear, the genetic predisposition of the disease in concordance with additional environmental factors can be given as the most common cause of Graves' disease [18, 19]. The infiltration of the thyroid gland by autoreactive T and B cells synthesis of cytokines results in producing TSH-receptor Ab. The production of auto-antibodies and the preexistence of genetic predisposition of Graves' along with external factors including a recurring infection, stress, smoking, or oral iodine results in Graves' mediated hyperthyroidism. The most common first-line therapy includes antithyroid drugs (ATD) [20, 21]. The lower liver toxicity makes thiamazole as most preferred ATD. The suboptimal remission rate limits the use of thiamazole therapy and offers the use of radioiodine therapy as primary treatment. Carbimazole and its active metabolite such as propylthiouracil (PTU) and methimazole (MMI) are other commonly used ATD for Graves'.

4.2 Thyroiditis (Hashimoto's disease)

Hashimoto thyroiditis is presented as an autoimmune disease that results from the self-destruction of thyroid cells by auto-antibody-mediated immune responses [22].

Progressive fibrosis resulting from damaged thyroid tissue by antithyroid antibodies is the most common pathology of Hashimoto's disease. Based on the pathology Hashimoto's can also be termed as chronic lymphocytic thyroiditis or autoimmune thyroiditis. Hashimoto's disease is most prevalent among women than men, particularly among women aged between 30 and 50 years [23]. Diagnosis remains a constraint in Hashimoto's as it still takes time even after the disease progression. Monitoring elevated levels of antithyroid peroxidase along with depleted levels of free thyroxine and elevated TSH is the most common diagnostic method [24]. Levothyroxine is the most common medication which acts by converting T4 to T3, the active form of thyroid hormone [25].

4.3 Thyrotoxicosis

The physiological malfunctions in the expression of excessive levels of thyroid hormones are characterized as thyrotoxicosis. Thyrotoxicosis refers to the release of excess thyroid hormone resulting from the rapid distraction of thyroid tissue and it is not associated with hyperfunction of the thyroid gland [26]. Viral infection or autoimmune malfunctions resulting in the inflammation of the thyroid gland is the prime cause of thyrotoxicosis [27]. High levels of circulating thyroid hormones exhibit a direct inotropic effect by increasing α- to β-myosin heavy chain expression which affects cardiac contraction. Increased appetite, heat intolerance, and increased basal metabolic rate results in metabolism and increased food intake [28, 29]. Based on the degree of the increased rate of metabolism, nutritional deficiency and chronic caloric inadequacy ensue. The increased basal metabolic rate results in increased synthesis and degradation of the protein. Increased protein metabolism results in severe thyrotoxicosis and a radical decrease in net protein content can be evidenced by muscle wasting, proximal muscle weakness, and loss of weight [30].

4.4 Toxic nodular goiter

Toxic nodular goiter is a hormonally heterogeneous disorder, goiter is a multinodular hyperthyroidism characterized by multifunctional thyroid nodules with normal, increased, or decreased thyroid hormone production [31]. The functional heterogenicity of normal follicular cells through genetic factors and also through accruing new inheritable qualities by replicating thyroid cells are the two major primary factors of nodular goiter [32]. Secondary factors include external aspects such as smoking, stress, high levels of TSH, pharmaceutical agents, TSF (IGF-1), and other exogenous factors. Iodine plays a pivotal role development of nodular goiters. Iodine deficiency results in hyperplasia with increased TSH levels, with raise in iodine to a normal level hyperplasia, go into the resting phase [33]. These physiological alterations result in the development of diffuse hyperplasia with a higher risk of developing uni-nodule or multi-nodular goiter. Toxic multinodular goiter exhibits characteristic precursors such as single toxic adenomas or nontoxic multinodular goiter. The other complications include congestive heart failure, rapid heart rate, and atrial fibrillation, which might also result in osteoporosis [34].

5. Causes of hyperthyroidism

Hyperthyroidism is a multifactorial hormonal disorder that varies according to the patient's age, degree of hormone synthesis, the incidence of similar health conditions, and extent of the illness. The clinical presentation of hyperthyroidism differentiates with each of the conditions given above [35]. Grave's disease and thyroiditis are the most common causes of hyperthyroidism. Grave's is commonly characterized as an autoimmune disease with an overproduction of thyroid hormone and this can be inherited or mostly associated with other autoimmune diseases. Thyroiditis is also an autoimmune condition resulting from inflammation of the thyroid gland [36]. An onset of thyrotoxic symptoms results from a hormone leak from the inflamed gland in subacute thyroiditis. Lymphocytic thyroiditis results from transient inflammatory causes and is difficult to distinguish from Graves at the early acute stage.

Various other factors influence the cause of hyperthyroidism which includes, but not limited to, such as excess thyroid hormone supplementation, iodine-induced hyperthyroidism, noncancerous tumor of the pituitary gland, and drugs associated with hyperthyroidism.

5.1 Exogenous thyroid hormone (acute or chronic)

The excessive intake of liothyronine, levothyroxine, or desiccated thyroid either intentionally or inadvertent may result in exogenous hyperthyroidism. Prevalence of exogenous hyperthyroidism is more common in elderly people than endogenous hyperthyroidism due to an intentional overdose of thyroid hormone [37]. Levothyroxine is the most common suppressive dose of thyroxine administered to treat patients with goiter and to suppress tumor growth. Drugs used for treating depression, infertility, and obesity were also known to cause exogenous hyperthyroidism. Overdose of thyroid hormones may result in bone loss, cardiac dysfunction, and myocardial infarction. Exogenous hyperthyroidism typically exhibits symptoms of thyrotoxicosis [38, 39].

5.2 Iodine-induced hyperthyroidism

Iodine-induced hyperthyroidism was first stated in 1821 and has been recurrently observed in patients when introduced to iodine in iodine-deficient areas. It was also observed in patients without a history of thyroid disease in iodine-sufficient areas. The disorder has been reported later in relatively low iodine intakes regions such as western Europe and regions with iodine-deficient goiter. Iodine-induced hyperthyroidism has been reported in iodine-sufficient areas such as the United States where iodine intake was far above the minimum daily requirement (50 to 100μg). The syndrome was commonly reported in iodine-sufficient areas without any other sign of thyroid diseases. This might result from pharmacological doses of iodine from common drugs such as Betadine, Iodo-Niacin, amiodarone, and various other radiographic dyes. Globally 800 million people are at risk of iodine deficiency (ID) and related disorders. Iodine supplementation is the most preventable approach to eliminating the risk of ID disorders. The term iodide refers to the biological form of the free element (inorganic), while iodine includes both inorganic iodides (I-) and iodine covalently bound to tyrosine [40]. The thyroid adopts several mechanisms to compensate for the iodine deficiency and to maintain sufficient thyroid production. Prolonged compensatory mechanisms result in the development of multifunctional autonomous growth and function of the thyroid with induced mutation of TSH receptors by harboring scattered cell clones [12, 41]. A high prevalence of multinodular goiter and nodular hyperthyroidism may be associated with mild prolonged ID (**Figure 1**) [42].

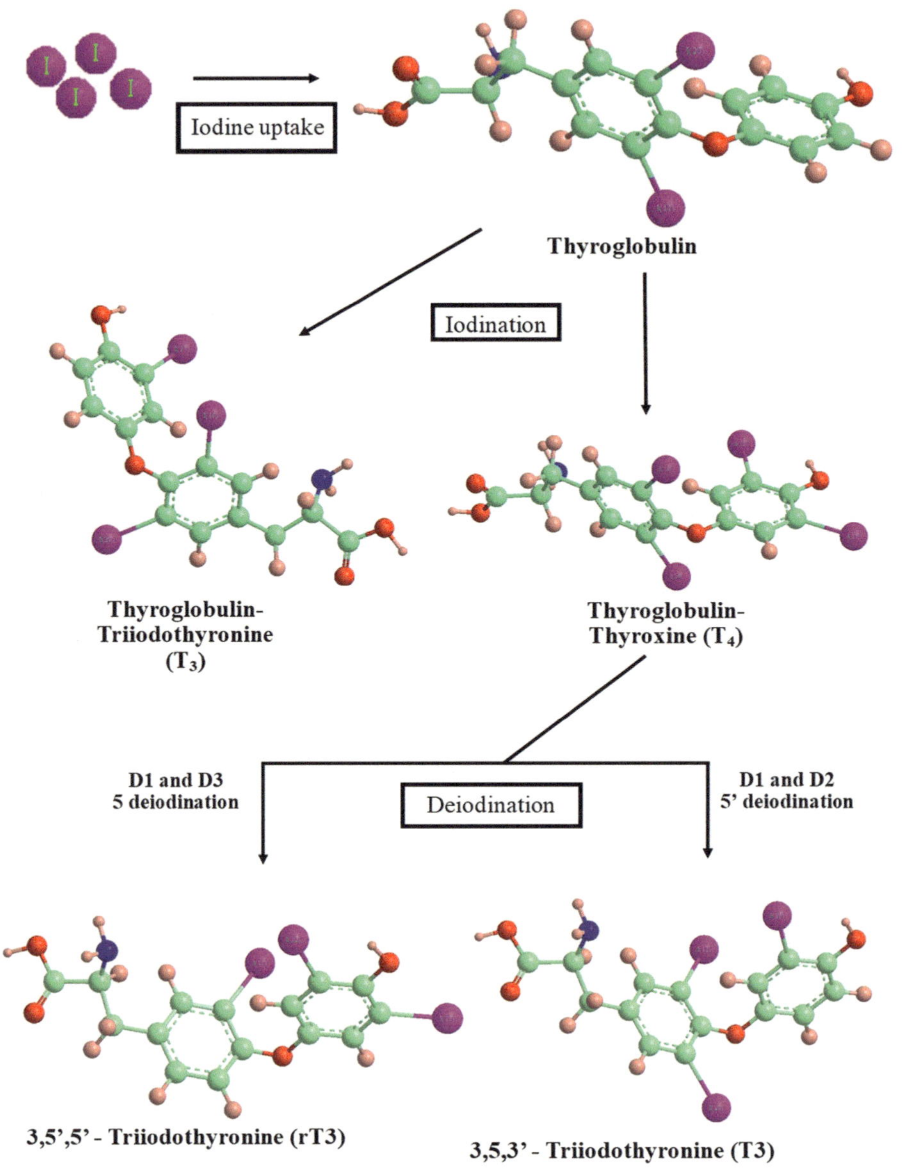

Figure 1.
Metabolic pathway of thyroid iodination and deiodination mediated by iodine deiodinases.

5.3 Noncancerous tumors of the pituitary gland

Thyrotroph adenomas are pituitary tumors that induce overproduction of thyroid-stimulating hormone resulting in hyperthyroidism. Among pituitary adenomas, thyrotropic adenomas account for less than 1% and are a rare cause of hyperthyroidism [43]. Pituitary adenomas are mostly benign and localized in the pituitary gland. Tumors spread to nearby tissues by expansion or invasion of their surroundings or tissue displacement and usually do not spread to other body parts [31]. TSH- secreting adenomas widely produce TSH (72%) alone where in certain cases, elevated secretion of TSH by adenomas results in activating various other hormones such as gonadotrophins, prolactinoma, and growth hormone which results in various physiological functioning of the brain by affecting cavernous sinus. Most of the thyroid-adenomas are macroadenomas (<10 mm) [44]. Hyperthyroidism along with thyrotroph adenomas are frequently associated with loss of vision, headache, visual defects, and loss of anterior pituitary functioning. Atrial fibrillation, thyrotoxic failure, and vertebral fracture are the few deleterious effects of thyrotroph adenomas [45].

5.4 Drug-associated hyperthyroidism

Drug-associated hyperthyroidism is commonly referred to as factitious hyperthyroidism resulting from inappropriate intake of thyroid hormones. Molecular-targeted agents, thyroid hormone, interferon, and amiodarone are the most common drugs associated with hyperthyroidism [45]. Amiodarone is a common drug used to treat heart rhythm disorder. The high iodine content of the drug accelerates the thyroid gland to secrete excessive amounts of thyroid hormones [46]. Alemtuzumab an anti-cancerous drug induces hyperthyroidism in patients by producing auto-antibodies against the thyroid gland and resulting in the development of Graves' disease. Another cancer drug PD-1 inhibitor used in cancer immunotherapy to boost the body's innate immune system results in the development of hyperthyroidism in patients by producing antibodies against thyroid hormones [47]. Highly active antiretroviral therapies, lithium, tyrosine kinase, and interferon α are other pharmaceutical compounds associated with drug-induced hyperthyroidism [48].

6. Micronutrients in hyperthyroidism

Nutritional factors are closely associated with regular physiological activities and optimal metabolic functioning. Dietary micronutrients are one of the predominant sources of essential micronutrients such as vitamins, minerals, trace elements, and amino acids [49]. Deficiency in these micronutrients results in great health concerns and according to the WHO, around 2 billion people are affected by micronutrient deficiency-related health disorders. Micronutrients mediate optimal metabolic functioning through the production of hormones, enzymes, and various biomolecules for optimal growth and development [50]. Despite being required in a small amount, a sensible deficiency of micronutrients results in detrimental effects on various physiological functioning such as regulating membrane permeability, enzymatic reactions, etc. [51]. Nutritional alterations are highly related to thyroid dysfunctions as the normal functioning of the thyroid is derived from optimal supplementation of various essential micronutrients.

The role of iodine and selenium in optimal production and proper metabolism of the thyroid is remarkable. Selenium-containing deiodinases play a pivotal role in the conversion of circulating T4 into physiologically active thyroid. The affinity of selenium-containing deiodinases toward specific receptors allows them to bind to receptors in nuclei, which in turn regulate gene expression. Selenium exists in the form of selenoproteins as functionally active. Glutathione peroxidase (GPX) and iodothyronine deiodinase are the two major enzymes with selenocysteine as an integral protein. Deiodinases generally exist in three forms, where 5′DII mediates the conversion of active thyroid hormone T3 from prohormone T4 and 5′DI catalyzes the degradation of rT3. The selenocysteine-containing deiodinase is involved in the feedback and inactivates both thyroid hormones T4 and T3. Selenocysteine containing GPX protects the thyroid tissues from oxidative damage caused by hydrogen peroxide during the synthesis of thyroid hormone. The precursor of selenocysteine, monoselenium is also involved in the cellular defense mechanism.

The efficacy of iodine can be improved by supplementation of vitamin A, which results in vitamin A-mediated TSH-β suppression. The patients with severe iodine deficiency were observed with increased levels of TSH, thyroglobulin, and goiter size due to a deficiency of vitamin A [52]. Fluorine inhibits iodine transport and exhibits an anti-thyroid effect. Dietary intake of fluorine results in severe iodine deficiency and at higher concentrations, it might lead to goitrogenic [53]. The iodine transportation to the thyroid gland is inhibited by bromine, which results in physiological changes in the cellular architecture and affects the thyroid secretions [54]. Cobalt at higher concentrations results in goiter and affects thyroid hormone production, whereas cobalt deficiency reduces T3 levels. The function of selenium in thyroid functioning is well-studied in iodine transport [55]. Metal ions like cadmium, zinc, mercury, and rubidium tend to mimic the role of selenium or impart with selenium in iodine transport. Where these metals have various negative effects on thyroid functioning, as cadmium in rats has proven to increase levels of T3 and T4, and it also affects the activity of hepatic D1 [56]. Rubidium has been reported with inducing goiter in rats. Calcium has been reported to interfere with thyroid functioning, where excess dietary calcium results in goiter and is associated with low iodine clearance. Calcium also inhibits thyroxine adsorption [57, 58]. Asparagine and serine have been found to be positively correlated with the expression of TSH. Synthesis of T4 and FT4 were correlated with certain amino acids namely valine, leucine, and arginine, and the same was reported by Krishnamurthy *et al.*, 2021.

7. Antinuclear antibodies (ANA) in early diagnosis of hyperthyroidism

Among the spectrum of autoimmune diseases, autoimmune thyroid diseases are the most common and are frequently associated with various organ-specific and non-organ-specific autoimmune disorders. Ani-thyroid peroxidase (Anti-TPO) and anti-thyroglobulin (Anti-Tg) are common markers of AITD. The prevalence of these anti-nuclear antibodies has been widely reported in AITD adult patients. ANA and other extractable antibodies are identified as novel diagnostic markers for predicting various autoimmune diseases. Over 90% of the patients with a multifactorial autoimmune disease such as systemic lupus erythematosus was detected with ANA. Various cross-sectional studies have reported the presence of ANA in healthy populations. A cross-sectional study by Satoh et al. [59] on 4754 individuals above 12 years reported the prevalence of ANA in 13.8% of the population. Another study by Hilário et al. [60] on healthy children reported the prevalence of ANA in 12.6% of the population. The rationale for the occurrence of these ANA remains unclear, but the assessment of these autoantibodies can be an early predictor of future autoimmune disorders.

Graves' disease and chronic lymphocytic thyroiditis are the most common organ-specific autoimmune disorders resulting from lymphocytic infiltration of autoantibodies and thyroid hormones. A retrospective analysis by Siriwardhane et al. [61] evaluated the association of thyroid hormones TSH, FT4, and anti-TPO antibodies and anti-Tg. In this study, the presence of ANA and anti-ENA were evaluated in subjects with systemic autoimmune disease markers such as thyroid, anti-TPO, and anti-Tg. They reported a strong prevalence of ANA in 20.4% of thyroid positive subjects,

18.0%, and 17.6% in anti-TPO and anti-Tg positive subjects respectively. In their retrospective study, they exhibited a strong association between ATID markers and systemic autoimmune markers and the prevalence of anti-TPO and ANA and anti-ENA as specific markers for autoimmune thyroid disorders. This also suggests that periodical evaluation of ANA and other autoimmune antibodies would assist in the early detection of autoimmunity among individuals who have anti-TPO antibodies.

8. Hyperthyroidism in human reproductive health

Thyroid hormones are vital endocrine enzymes in maintaining regular metabolism and healthy reduction in both males and females. Alterations in thyroid synthesis have adverse effects on reproductive health. Sex steroids and sex-hormone-binding globulins are the prime metabolites associated with thyroid disorders. Both hyperthyroidism and hypothyroidism have considerable effects on reproductive health, whereas overactive thyroid is associated with various reproductive dysfunctions. In males, hyperactive thyroid results in impaired sexual behavior, a decrease in morphologically normal sperm, reduction in sperm motility and count. In females, thyroid imbalance mainly results in menstrual disturbances and reduced fertility. Hyperthyroidism is also associated with polymenorrhea and hypomenorrhea. A sharp increase in estrogen levels can be observed in hyperthyroid women and levels of SHBG were also found to increase. The production rate of testosterone and androstenedione was found to significantly increase in hyperthyroid women along with changes in androgen metabolism.

Hyperthyroidism in men is primarily characterized by elevated levels of SHBG resulting in increased levels of circulating total testosterone. Studies have reported that concentrations of free testosterone remain stable whereas the circulating levels of bioavailable testosterone were found to be depleted. Both total and free estradiol concentrations were found to decrease in hyperthyroid subjects. Overactive thyroid had adverse effects on semen quality, a study by Clyde et al. reported marked oligospermia resulting in low motility in two out of three hyperthyroid patients, where one was reported with low sperm count. A similar study by Kidd et al. in five hyperthyroid patients reported low sperm counts in all subjects.

A comprehensive retrospective analysis by Siriwardhane et al. analyzed the effects of altered thyroid hormones on vital sex hormones. The study with 15,043 subjects between the reproductive age of 15–49 years reported elevated levels of total testosterone and SHBG in hyperthyroid women. Anti-TPO seropositive women reported elevated testosterone and low cortisol. Whereas hyperthyroid men were reported with low DHEA-S and elevated estradiol, FSH, and prolactin. The study reported an inverse direction of SHBG levels in hyperthyroid and hypothyroid subjects in women. The positive correlation between SHBG with thyroid hormones FT3 and FT4 has been reported in various studies. The reduction in the metabolic clearance rate of testosterone due to the increased affinity between SHBG and testosterone increases the circulating levels of testosterone. This study also suggested that thyroid hormones could activate steroidogenesis in hyperthyroid patients resulting in increased levels of DHEA-S.

9. Role of anti-TPO in early detection of hyperthyroidism

Thyroid-specific auto-immune disorders are the second most organ-specific autoimmune disorder next to rheumatoid arthritis. Graves' disease and Hashimoto's thyroiditis are the most common thyroid-specific auto-immune disease. The pathogenesis of AITD includes various environmental and genetic factors. Anti-thyroid peroxidase is an antibody that synthesizes against a transmembrane of thyrocyte and is related to the levels of TSH which can be used to predict thyroid abnormalities. Over 90% of the cases with Hashimoto's thyroiditis and 80% of cases with Graves' disease are reported with the presence of anti-TPO. Anti-TPO antibodies in AITD subjects act as competitive inhibitors of thyroid activity and destroy thyrocytes. Anti-TPO antibodies highly belong to the IgG1 and IgG4 class of autoantibodies. Anti-TPO is an effective indicator of thyroid disease and also could indicate oxidative stress, advanced glycation, and oxygen metabolites in blood. Several studies have reported the presence of anti-TPO in Graves' disease, the recurrence of Graves' disease can be predicted by systemic evaluation of anti-TPO after anti-thyroid treatment [62].

A retrospective analysis by siriwardhane et al. reported the prevalence of anti-TPO as a selective marker for the early prediction of thyroid diseases. The results revealed the presence of anti-TPO prior to the onset of thyroid disease in both hyperthyroid and hypothyroid patients. The study also reported the occurrence of anti-TPO antibodies lacking any alterations in thyroid hormone levels. The study also reported that the anti-Tg antibody is a less specific marker for thyroid disease. A similar study by Hutfless et al. reported the prevalence of anti-TPO and anti-Tg antibodies 7 years prior to the diagnosis of Hashimoto's and Graves' disease. In summary, the thyroid system has a complex interplay with various factors including nutrition, autoimmunity, and reproductive function. Though some of these associations have been highlighted in the past decades, novel biochemistry and better diagnostic capabilities are unraveling novel associations that are leading to a more nuanced understanding of thyroid functions. This chapter explores some of these novel associations and sheds light on exciting outcomes that may arise in the years to come.

Acknowledgments

We acknowledge Vibrant America LLC for supporting this research.

Conflict of interest

The authors declare no conflict of interest.

Author details

Hari Krishnan Krishnamurthy[1*†], Swarnkumar Reddy[2†], Vasanth Jayaraman[1], Karthik Krishna[1], Karenah E. Rajasekaran[2], Tianhao Wang[1], Kang Bei[1] and John J. Rajasekaran[1*]

1 Vibrant Sciences LLC., San Carlos, CA, United States of America

2 Vibrant America LLC., San Carlos, CA, United States of America

*Address all correspondence to: hari@vibrantsci.com and jjrajasekaran@vibrantsci.com

†These authors are joint senior authors on this work.

References

[1] Kravets I. Hyperthyroidism: Diagnosis and treatment. American Family Physician. 2016;**93**(5):363-370

[2] Taurog A. Hormone synthesis: Thyroid iodine metabolism. In: Werner and Ingbar's the Thyroid. Lippincott-Raven; 2000. pp. 61-85

[3] Rousset B, Dupuy C, Miot F, Dumont J. Thyroid hormone synthesis and secretion. Endotext. 2015;**2000**:2015

[4] Arthur JR, Beckett GJ. Thyroid function. British Medical Bulletin. 1999;**55**(3):658-668

[5] Tata JR, Widnell CC. Ribonucleic acid synthesis during the early action of thyroid hormones. Biochemical Journal. 1966;**98**(2):604

[6] Godswill AG, Somtochukwu IV, Ikechukwu AO, Kate EC. Health benefits of micronutrients (vitamins and minerals) and their associated deficiency diseases: A systematic review. International Journal of Food Sciences. 2020;**3**(1):1-32

[7] Kopp P. Human genome and diseases: Review the TSH receptor and its role in thyroid disease. Cellular and Molecular Life Sciences CMLS. 2001;**58**(9):1301-1322

[8] Galofré JC, Díez JJ, Cooper DS. Thyroid dysfunction in the era of precision medicine. Endocrinología y Nutrición (English Edition). 2016;**63**(7):354-363

[9] Siriwardhane T, Krishna K, Song Q, Ranganathan V, Jayaraman V, Wang T, et al. Human reproductive health in relation to thyroid alterations. Health. 2019;**11**(08):1095

[10] Lewis W. Hyperthyroidism and associated pathology. The Journal of Nervous and Mental Disease. 1931;**74**(1):102

[11] Mathew P, Rawla P. Hyperthyroidism. StatPearls; 2022

[12] Delange F, De Benoist B, Alnwick D. Risks of iodine-induced hyperthyroidism after correction of iodine deficiency by iodized salt. Thyroid. 1999;**9**(6):545-556

[13] Leung AM, Braverman LE. Iodine-induced thyroid dysfunction. Current Opinion in Endocrinology, Diabetes, and Obesity. 2012;**19**(5):414

[14] van Hoek I, Hesta M, Biourge V. A critical review of food-associated factors proposed in the etiology of feline hyperthyroidism. Journal of Feline Medicine and Surgery. 2015;**17**(10):837-847

[15] Sajjadi-Jazi SM, Sharifi F, Varmaghani M, Meybodi HA, Farzadfar F, Larijani B. Epidemiology of hyperthyroidism in Iran: A systematic review and meta-analysis. Journal of Diabetes & Metabolic Disorders. 2018;**17**(2):345-355

[16] Siegel RD, Lee SL. Toxic nodular goiter: Toxic adenoma and toxic multinodular goiter. Endocrinology and Metabolism Clinics of North America. 1998;**27**(1):151-168

[17] Weetman AP. Graves' disease. New England Journal of Medicine. 2000;**343**(17):1236-1248

[18] Brent GA. Graves' disease. New England Journal of Medicine. 2008;**358**(24):2594-2605

[19] Burch HB, Cooper DS. Management of Graves disease: A review. JAMA. 2015;**314**(23):2544-2554

[20] Bartalena L. Diagnosis and management of graves disease: A global overview. Nature Reviews Endocrinology. 2013;**9**(12):724-734

[21] Prummel MF, Wiersinga WM. Smoking and risk of Graves' disease. JAMA. 1993;**269**(4):479-482

[22] Pearce EN, Farwell AP, Braverman LE. Thyroiditis. New England Journal of Medicine. 2003;**348**(26):2646-2655

[23] Boelaert K, Newby PR, Simmonds MJ, Holder RL, Carr-Smith JD, Heward JM, et al. Prevalence and relative risk of other autoimmune diseases in subjects with autoimmune thyroid disease. The American Journal of Medicine. 2010;**123**(2):183-1e1

[24] Demirbilek HÜSEYİN, Kandemir NURGÜN, Gonc EN, Ozon A, Alikasifoglu A, Yordam NURŞEN. Hashimoto's thyroiditis in children and adolescents: A retrospective study on clinical, epidemiological and laboratory properties of the disease. Journal of Pediatric Endocrinology and Metabolism. 2007;**20**(11):1199-1206

[25] Ehlers M, Schott M. Hashimoto's thyroiditis and papillary thyroid cancer: Are they immunologically linked? Trends in Endocrinology & Metabolism. 2014;**25**(12):656-664

[26] Nayak B, Burman K. Thyrotoxicosis and thyroid storm. Endocrinology and Metabolism Clinics. 2006;**35**(4):663-686

[27] Lania A, Sandri MT, Cellini M, Mirani M, Lavezzi E, Mazziotti G. Thyrotoxicosis in patients with COVID-19: The THYRCOV study. European Journal of Endocrinology. 2020;**183**(4):381-387

[28] Devereaux D, Tewelde SZ. Hyperthyroidism and thyrotoxicosis. Emergency medicine. Clinics. 2014;**32**(2):277-292

[29] Blick C, Nguyen M, Jialal I. Thyrotoxicosis. StatPearls Publishing; 2021

[30] Blick C, Schreyer KE. Gestational trophoblastic disease-induced thyroid storm. Clinical Practice and Cases in Emergency Medicine. 2019;**3**(4):409

[31] Aksoy DY, Gedik A, Cinar N, Soylemezoglu F, Berker M, Gurlek OA. Thyrotropinoma and multinodular goiter: A diagnostic challenge for hyperthyroidism. Journal of Research in Medical Sciences: The Official Journal of Isfahan University of Medical Sciences. 2013;**18**(11):1008

[32] Khalid N, Can AS. Plummer Disease. Treasure Island (FL): StatPearls Publishing 2021

[33] Mahajan, A., Ghaznavi, S.A., Lithgow, K. and Paschke, R., 2019. Toxic Multinodular Goiter

[34] Faggiano A, Del Prete M, Marciello F, Marotta V, Ramundo V, Colao A. Thyroid diseases in elderly. Minerva Endocrinologica. 2011;**36**(3):211-231

[35] De Leo S, Lee SY. Lewis E Braverman published in final edited form as. Lancet. 2016;**388**(10047):906-918

[36] LaFranchi S. Thyroiditis and acquired hypothyroidism. Pediatric Annals. 1992;**21**(1):29-39

[37] Batrinos ML. The problem of exogenous subclinical hyperthyroidism. Hormones Athens. 2006;**5**(2):119

[38] Toft AD. Subclinical hyperthyroidism. New England Journal of Medicine. 2001;**345**(7):512-516

[39] Biondi B, Palmieri EA, Klain M, Schlumberger M, Filetti S, Lombardi G. Subclinical hyperthyroidism: Clinical features and treatment options. European Journal of Endocrinology. 2005;**152**(1):1-9

[40] Roti E, Uberti ED. Iodine excess and hyperthyroidism. Thyroid. 2001;**11**(5):493-500

[41] Yang F, Teng W, Shan Z, Guan H, Li Y, Jin Y, et al. Epidemiological survey on the relationship between different iodine intakes and the prevalence of hyperthyroidism. European Journal of Endocrinology. 2002;**146**(5):613-618

[42] Martin FIR, Tress BW, Colman PG, Deam DR. Iodine-induced hyperthyroidism due to nonionic contrast radiography in the elderly. The American Journal of Medicine. 1993;**95**(1):78-82

[43] Beck-Peccoz P, Persani L, Mantovani S, Cortelazzi D, Asteria C. Thyrotropin-secreting pituitary adenomas. Metabolism. 1996;**45**:75-78

[44] Beck-Peccoz P, Persani L, Mannavola D, Campi I. TSH-secreting adenomas. Best Practice & Research Clinical Endocrinology & Metabolism. 2009;**23**(5):597-606

[45] Buchfelder M, Fahlbusch R. Thyrotroph adenomas. In: Diagnosis and Management of Pituitary Tumors. Totowa, NJ: Humana Press; 2001. pp. 333-342

[46] Atkins P, Cohen SB, Phillips BJ. Drug therapy for hyperthyroidism in pregnancy. Drug Safety. 2000;**23**(3):229-244

[47] Abraham P, Avenell A, Park CM, Watson WA, Bevan JS. A systematic review of drug therapy for graves' hyperthyroidism. European Journal of Endocrinology. 2005;**153**(4):489-498

[48] Ekiz Bilir B, Soysal Atile N, Kirkizlar O, Kömürcü Y, Akpinar S, Sezer A, et al. Effectiveness of preoperative plasmapheresis in a pregnancy complicated by hyperthyroidism and anti-thyroid drug-associated angioedema. Gynecological Endocrinology. 2013;**29**(5):508-510

[49] Bassuk SS, Manson JE. Epidemiological evidence for the role of physical activity in reducing risk of type 2 diabetes and cardiovascular disease. Journal of Applied Physiology. 2005;**2005**(3):1193-1204

[50] Hänsch R, Mendel RR. Physiological functions of mineral micronutrients (cu, Zn, Mn, Fe, Ni, Mo, B, cl). Current Opinion in Plant Biology. 2009;**12**(3):259-266

[51] Huskisson E, Maggini S, Ruf M. The influence of micronutrients on cognitive function and performance. Journal of International Medical Research. 2007;**35**(1):1-19

[52] Zimmermann MB, Jooste PL, Mabapa NS, Schoeman S, Biebinger R, Mushaphi LF, et al. Vitamin A supplementation in iodine-deficient African children decreases thyrotropin stimulation of the thyroid and reduces the goiter rate. The American Journal of Clinical Nutrition. 2007;**86**(4):1040-1044

[53] Galletti PM, Joyet G. Effect of fluorine on thyroidal iodine metabolism in hyperthyroidism. The Journal of Clinical Endocrinology & Metabolism. 1958;**18**(10):1102-1110

[54] Velický J, TItlbach M, Dušková J, Vobecký M, Štrbák V, Raška I. Potassium bromide and the thyroid gland of the rat:

Morphology and immunohistochemistry, RIA and INAA analysis. Annals of Anatomy-Anatomischer Anzeiger. 1997;**179**(5):421-431

[55] Pimentel-Malaussena E, Roche M, Layrisse M. Treatment of eight cases of hyperthyroidism with cobaltous chloride. Journal of the American Medical Association. 1958;**167**(14):1719-1722

[56] Bach I, Braun S, Gati T, Kertai P, Sos J, Udvardy A. Effect of rubidium on the thyroid. In: Pitt-Rivers R, editor. Advances in Thyroid Research. New York: Pergamon Press; 1961

[57] Gupta P, Kar A. Role of ascorbic acid in cadmium-induced thyroid dysfunction and lipid peroxidation. In: Journal of Applied Toxicology: An International Forum Devoted to Research and Methods Emphasizing Direct Clinical, Industrial and Environmental Applications. Chichester: John Wiley & Sons, Ltd; 1998, September. pp. 317-320

[58] Paier B, Pavia MA Jr, Hansi C, Noli MI, Hagmüller K, Zaninovich AA. Cadmium inhibits the in vitro conversion of thyroxine to triiodothyronine in rat brown adipose tissue. Bulletin of Environmental Contamination and Toxicology. 1997;**59**(1):164-170

[59] Satoh M, Tanaka S, Ceribelli A, Calise SJ, Chan EK. A comprehensive overview on myositis-specific antibodies: New and old biomarkers in idiopathic inflammatory myopathy. Clinical Reviews in Allergy & Immunology. 2017;**52**:1-19

[60] Hilário MOE, Arnaldo LC, Campos RS, Teresa TM, Almeida G, Eduardo CAL. Frequency of antinuclear antibodies in healthy children and adolescents. Clinical Pediatrics. 2004;**43**(7):637-642

[61] Siriwardhane T, Krishna K, Ranganathan V, Jayaraman V, Wang T, Bei K, et al. Exploring systemic autoimmunity in thyroid disease subjects. Journal of Immunology Research. 2018;**2018**. Article ID 6895146

[62] Siriwardhane T, Krishna K, Ranganathan V, Jayaraman V, Wang T, Bei K, et al. Significance of anti-TPO as an early predictive marker in thyroid disease. Autoimmune Diseases. 2019;**2019**. Article ID 1684074

Chapter 8

Surgery for Primary Hyperparathyroidism without Leaving a Visible Scar

Elias Karakas and Stefan Schopf

Abstract

Surgery for primary hyperparathyroidism changed significantly during the past decades, since localization procedures have been developed and became more and more reliable. Like in thyroid surgery, minimally invasive techniques are widely used. Furthermore, remote access techniques have evolved in thyroid surgery with the aim of optimizing cosmetic results by avoiding a visible scar on the neck. Transoral Endoscopic access *via* the vestibular approach (TOEPVA) is the newest remote access technique, also feasible and safe in parathyroid surgery with optimum cosmetic results.

Keywords: transoral, parathyroid, surgery, feasibility, safety, cosmesis

1. Introduction

Since the first operation for primary hyperparathyroidism (pHPT) surgery has been safely performed *via* an anterior neck incision. A better understanding of the underlying causes for pHPT in combination with evolving and improving localization procedures surgical approaches changed from the bilateral cervical exploration *via* a cervical skin incision to more and more focused and minimally invasive approaches [1].

These focused approaches are nowadays considered as the new gold standard in localized pHPT [2].

In most patients, wound healing is without any problems, especially after a skin incision of less than 2 cm (**Figure 1**). However, a worldwide consideration of potential wound healing problems may lead to a more differentiated appraisal (**Figure 2**). In African countries, for example, the incidence of keloid development after skin incision is up to 15% and in some countries, a scar on the neck is historically related to a negative standing.

Also, in western countries, nearly 20% of patients will experience some feelings of self-consciousness years after open neck surgery. More than 10% will consider further treatments such as plastic surgery to their cervical scars [3]. The impact of a the cervical incision on the health-related quality of life (HRQOL) was found to be like the impact of vitiligo, psoriasis, or severe atopic dermatitis in one series [4, 5]. Foremost in the thyroid but also in parathyroid surgery remote access surgery has evolved with the aim to optimize cosmesis [6].

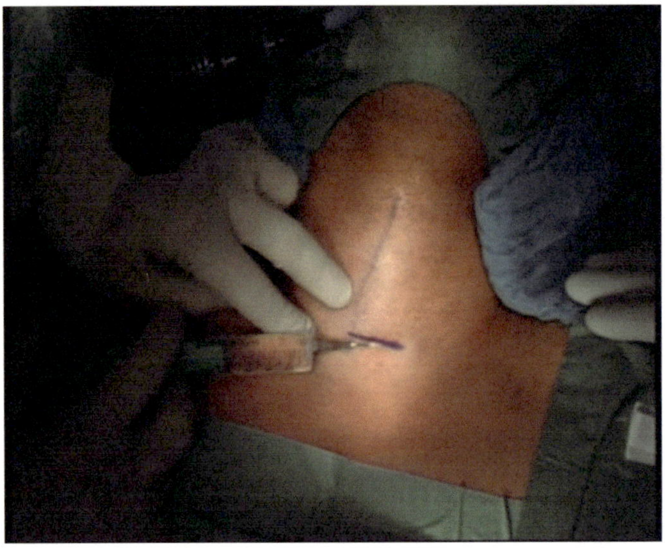

Figure 1.
Minimal almost 2 cm skin incision in focused parathyroid surgery.

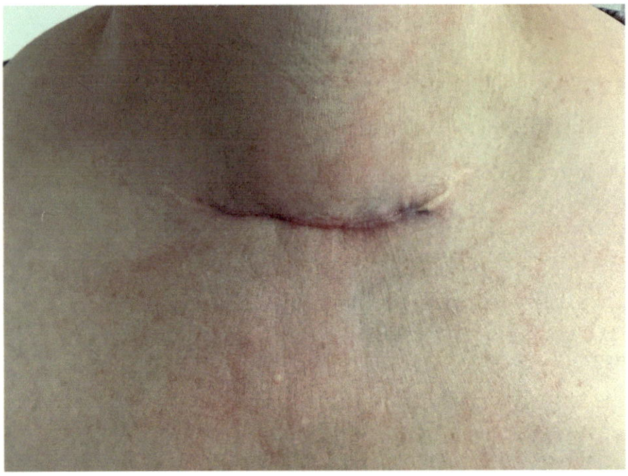

Figure 2.
Keloid in a small cervical scar.

Remote access surgery includes the areolar or axillary or combined areolar/axillary (ABBA) incisions and the retroauricular approach, which can effectively minimize the cosmetic burden on some patients. Improved cosmesis on one hand but unfamiliar dissection planes, longer routes to the central neck, and novel complications, on the other hand lead to further investigations focusing on the so-called natural orifice approaches. The emerging transoral thyroid and parathyroid vestibular approach—TOETVA in thyroid and TOEPVA in parathyroid surgery—was inspired by the idea to follow the embryologic thyroglossal duct. While feasibility was proven in substantial experimental and preclinical investigations by different study groups since 2006 and the first transoral parathyroid resection was done in 2010 [7], the clinical proof of concept was given by Anuwong, who published the first case series of 60 patients who underwent scarless thyroidectomy *via* the lower vestibule of the mouth with excellent outcomes [8]. This was followed by the first series of transoral transvestibular parathyroid operations with also promising results by Sasanakietkul et al. [9].

TOEPVA can be performed for select patients with localized primary hyperparathyroidism (HPT). Those without parathyroid adenoma localization, recurrent or persistent primary HPT, suspected multigland disease, secondary or tertiary HPT, family history of MEN, suspected parathyroid carcinoma, or previous central neck surgery or neck irradiation therapy should be excluded from consideration. Similar to TOETVA, the patient should also be highly motivated for a "scarless" approach.

2. TOEPVA: parathyroid surgery without leaving a visible scar

2.1 History of parathyroid surgery

Over more than 50 years bilateral cervical exploration (BCE) was the gold standard in parathyroid surgery. All parathyroids are visualized to resect the macroscopically enlarged gland [10]. BCE is associated with a more than 95% cure rate and minimal morbidity in experienced hands. In these times "the only localization that a patient needs who has primary hyperparathyroidism is the localization of an experienced surgeon!" [11]. Because primary HPT is a single gland disease in more than 80% and preoperative localization procedures have emerged and improved during the past decades minimally invasive procedures have been developed to minimize cervical skin incisions. These less invasive operations offer similar cure rates and result in equal complications compared to open surgery [12–14]. Minimally invasive parathyroidectomy leads to lower hospital costs, shorter length of stay, and equally high cure rates with low complication rates [15, 16].

2.2 Prerequisites, patients, and surgical technique

Surgeons interested in performing transoral parathyroid surgery should be well-experienced in parathyroid surgery. In addition, experience with laparoscopic instrumentation is beneficial. The transoral technique should be trained within cadaver courses meanwhile frequently offered in specialized centers. Subsequently, the first transoral operations in the clinical setting should ideally performed with the assistance of an experienced transoral surgeon. The suspected parathyroid gland should be safely detected in one, better two preoperative localization procedures.

The transoral procedure should safely be implemented in patients with small thyroid specimens and benign thyroid nodules <20 mm in diameter.

2.3 Postoperative recommendations

In case of recurrent laryngeal nerve palsy (RLNP), patients should be reevaluated 1 week and/or 4 weeks after surgery and, if necessary, logopedics should be initiated with reevaluation 3 and 6 months after surgery.

Potential paresthesia in the chin area and lower lip due to mental nerve injury should carefully be documented postoperatively during a hospital stay. In case of persistent paresthesia, patients should be reevaluated 3, 6, and 12 months after surgery. In addition, patients should be introduced to grimace and repeatedly activate their mimic muscles directly after surgery.

Serum Calcium (Ca) as well as parathyroid hormone (PTH) levels should be measured pre- and postoperatively on day one to prove the success of the operation. To exclude persistence Ca levels should be monitored for 6 months. In case of low vitamin D levels and potential bone involvement Ca and vitamin D should be provided.

3. TOEPVA technique step by step

3.1 Surgical technique

Patients are placed in a supine position with a slight neck extension (**Figure 3a**). The use of intraoperative nerve monitoring (IONM) is strongly recommended. The endotracheal tube provided with an electrode for IONM can easily be placed transorally. A transnasal tube placement is not necessary (**Figure 3b**).

The mucosa of the oral cavity should be cleansed with chlorhexidine solution. Afterward, three small incisions, 1–1.5 cm in the midline and 5 mm lateral right and left are made in the lower lip as close to the lip vermilion and as far away from the branches of the mental nerve as possible (**Figures 4a** and **b**).

Afterward, a subplatysmal space is created by hydro-dissection using an epinephrine-enriched saline solution injected with a Verress needle. The subplatysmal space is widened using a blunt dissector (**Figures 5a, b** and **c**).

Three trocars (originally one 10 mm and two 5 mm in diameter) are inserted through the midline and lateral incisions, followed by high-flow CO2 gas insufflation at a maximum pressure of 8 mmHg (**Figure 6**).

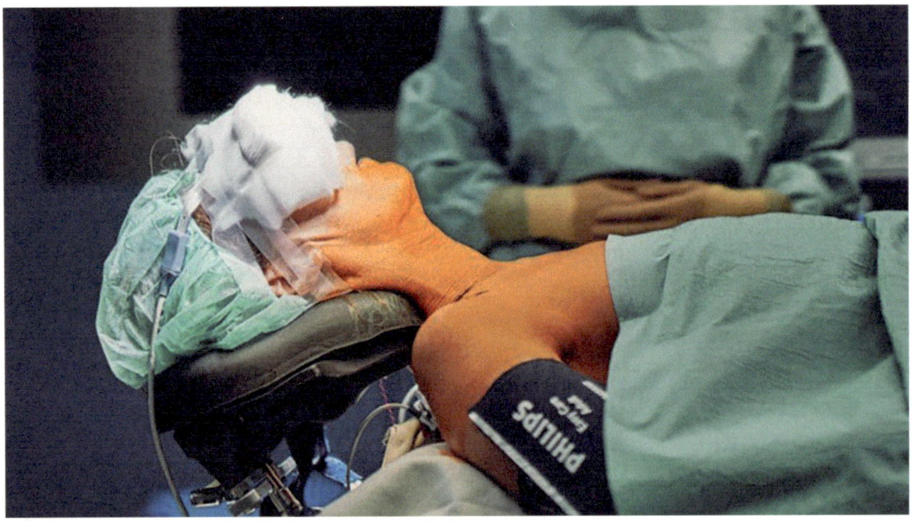

Figure 3a.
Patient's positioning with eye protection.

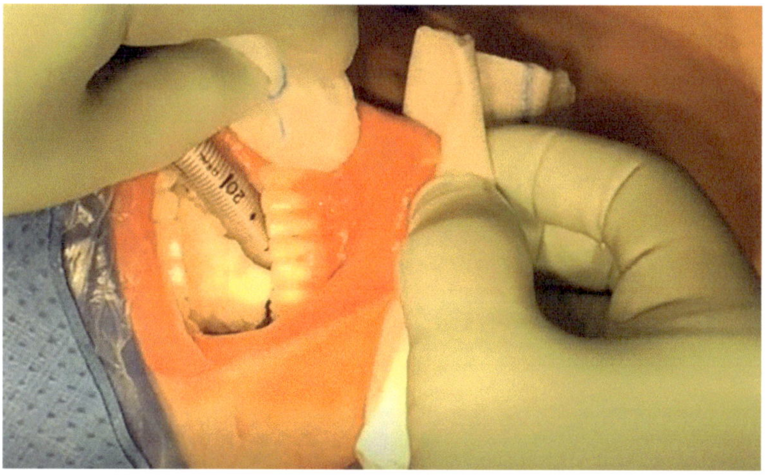

Figure 3b.
Transoral tube placement and disinfection of the mucosa.

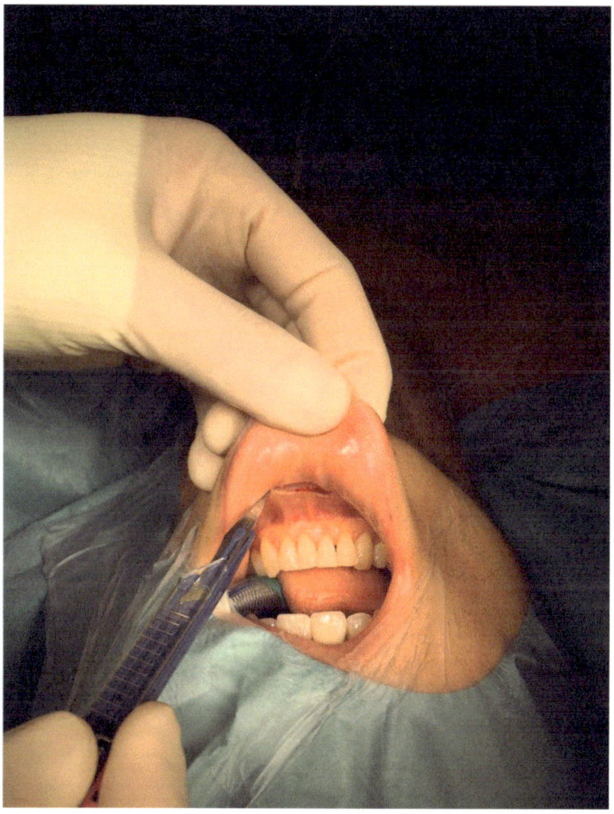

Figure 4a.
Midline incision close to the lip vermilion to avoid mental nerve injury.

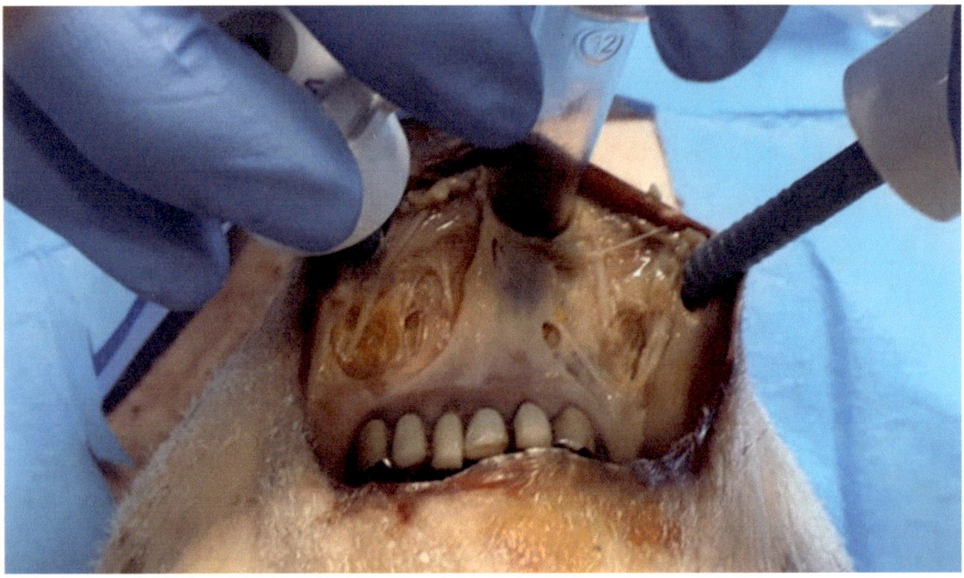

Figure 4b.
Cadaver study regarding trocar placement and mental nerve branches.

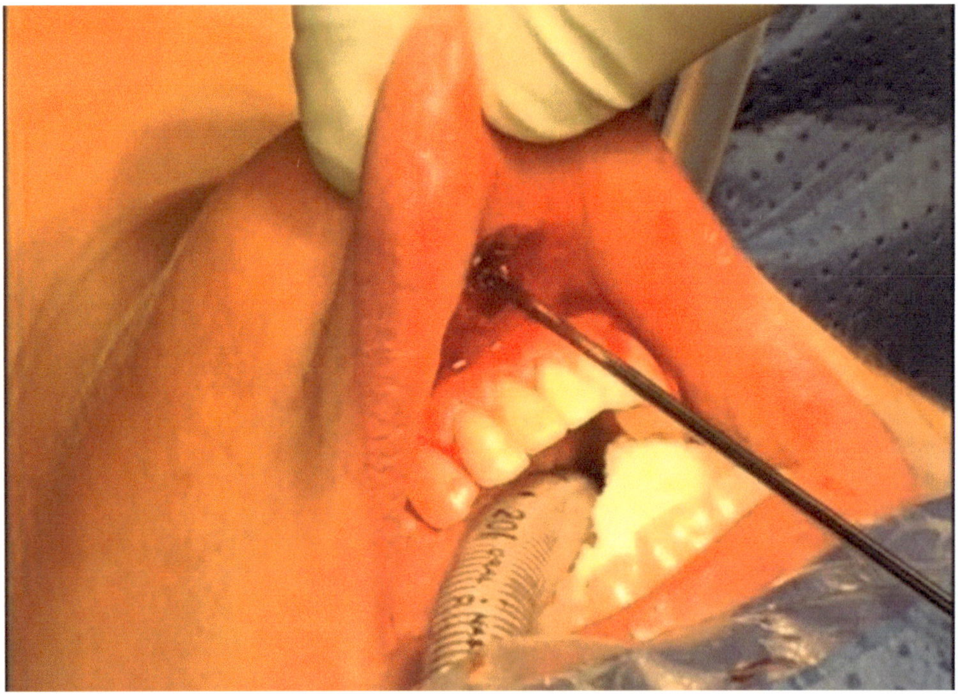

Figure 5a.
Application of epinephrine enriched saline solution with Verres needle to create an artificial subplatysmal space.

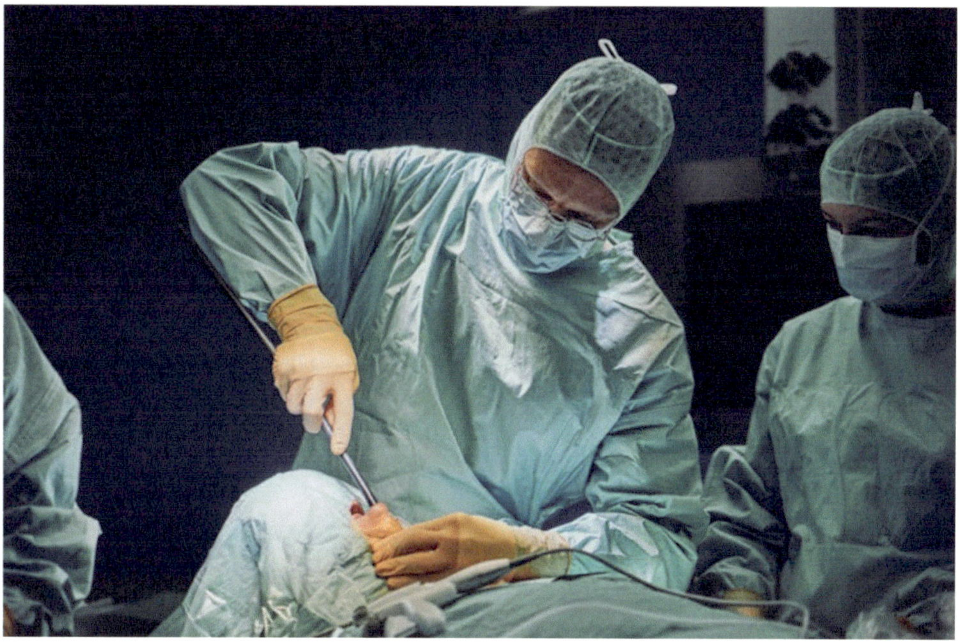

Figure 5b.
Blunt dissection of the artificial subplatysmal space.

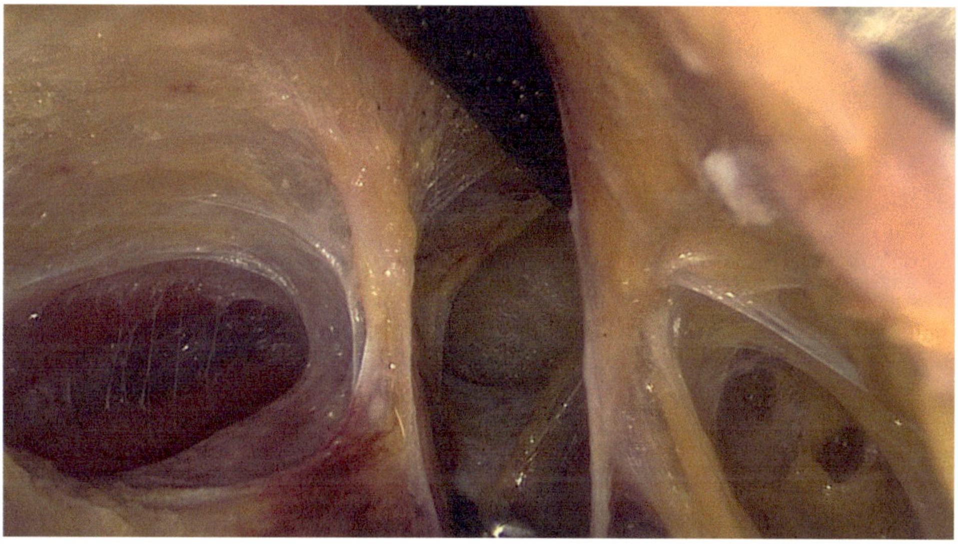

Figure 5c.
Artificial subplatysmal space.

Either a 5 mm or a 10 mm 30° full HD camera is used as well as conventional laparoscopic instruments. The subplatysmal working space reaches from the thyroid cartilage to the sternal notch and the medial border of both sternocleidomastoid muscles.

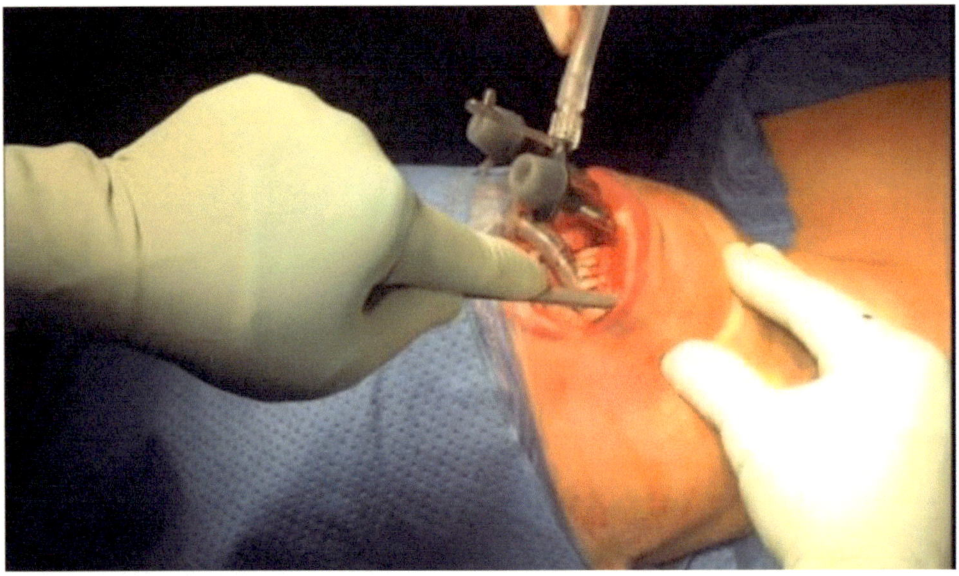

Figure 6.
Trocar placement—3 trocars 5 mm in the vestibulum oris.

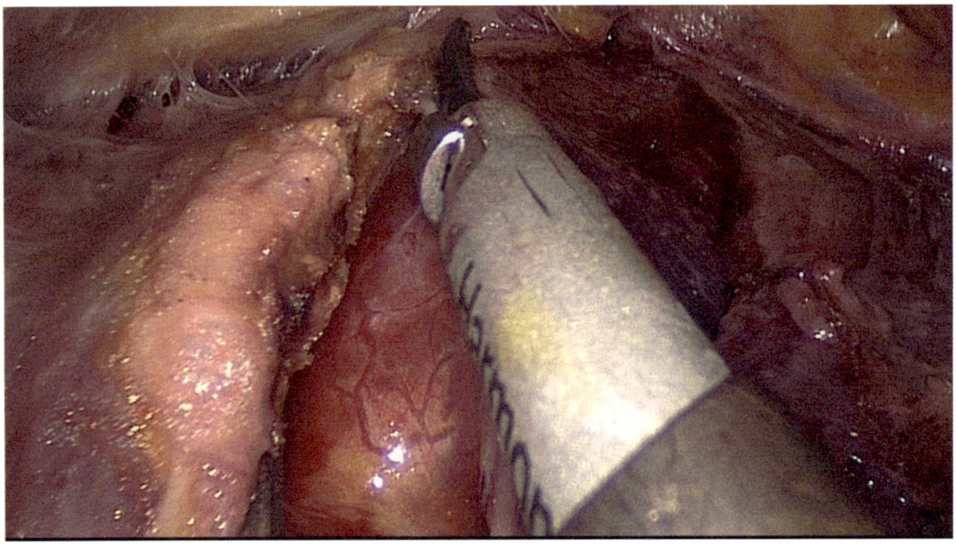

Figure 7.
Division of the strap muscles in the midline with a sealing device.

The strap muscles are divided in the midline and the lateral space of the assumed side will be dissected (**Figure 7**). In addition to gas insufflation two stitches are placed from outside to retract the strap muscles ventrally and laterally to optimize the working space (**Figure 8**).

Vessels should be selectively sealed with a thermal device. As in minimally invasive open surgery, the RLN does not routinely be visualized in case of a lower

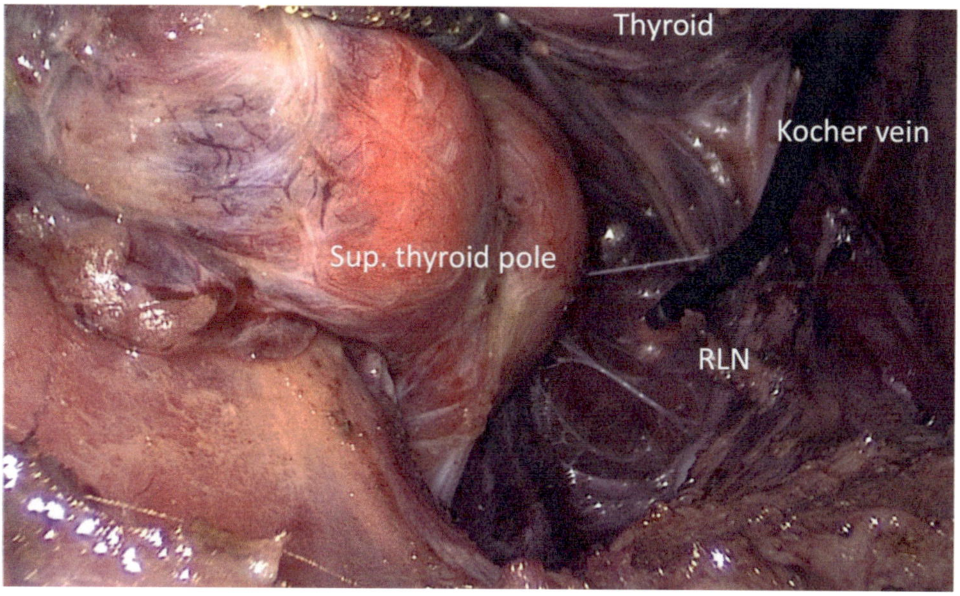

Figure 8.
Retracted muscles and lateral dissection.

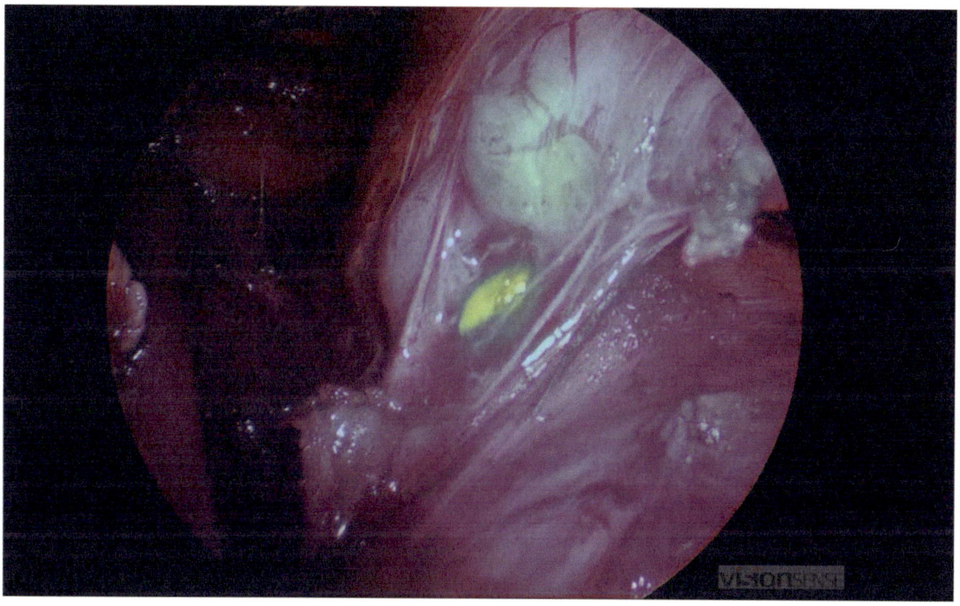

Figure 9.
Localization and identification of a parathyroid gland with indocyanine green fluorescent agent. (with courtesy of Prof. Philip Riss university hospital Vienna, Austria).

parathyroid adenoma. In addition, parathyroid glands can be visualized using fluorescent agents (**Figure 9**).

The resected parathyroid specimen is extracted through the midline trocar access.

Strap muscles are not adapted routinely at the end of the operation. Oral mucosa as well as retroauricular skin incision are closed using a 4/0 absorbable suture.

4. Conclusion

Transoral parathyroid surgery is feasible and save. As in conventional open minimal invasive surgery experience of the surgeon in parathyroid surgery and positive preoperative localization is essential.

Acknowledgements

We thank the EUROPEAN Study Group for Transoral Surgery, especially Prof. Philipp Riss and Prof. Christian Scheuba for providing figures regarding the use of fluorescend agents in transoral parathyroid surgery.

Conflict of interest

The authors declare no conflict of interest.

Author details

Elias Karakas[1] and Stefan Schopf[2*]

1 Hospital Maria Hilf, Alexianer GmbH, Krefeld, Germany

2 RoMed Hospital Bad Aibling, Germany

*Address all correspondence to: stefan.schopf@ro-med.de

References

[1] Miccoli P, Bendinelli C, Berti P, Vignali E, Pinchera A, Marcocci C. Video-assisted versus conventional parathyroidectomy in primary hyperparathyroidism: A prospective randomized study. Surgery. 1999;**126**(6):1117-1122

[2] Ahmadieh H, Kreidieh O, Akl EA, El-Hajj FG. Minimally invasive parathyroidectomy guided by intraoperative parathyroid hormone monitoring (IOPTH) and preoperative imaging versus bilateral neck exploration for primary hyperparathyroidism in adults. Cochrane Database of Systematic Reviews. 2020;(10). Art. No.: CD010787. DOI: 10.1002/14651858.CD010787.pub2

[3] Best AR, Shipchandler TZ, Cordes SR. Midcervical scar satisfaction in thyroidectomy patients. The Laryngoscope. 2017;**127**:1247-1252. DOI: 10.1002/lary.26177

[4] Choi Y, Lee JH, Kim YH, et al. Impact of postthyroidectomy scar on the quality of life of thyroid cancer patients. Annals of Dermatology. 2014;**26**:693-699. DOI: 10.5021/ad.2014.26.6.693

[5] Arora A, Swords C, Garas G, et al. The perception of scar cosmesis following thyroid and parathyroid surgery: A prospective cohort study. International Journal of Surgery. 2016;**25**:38-43. DOI: 10.1016/j.ijsu.2015.11.021

[6] Berber E, Bernet V, Fahey TJ 3rd, et al. American thyroid association statement on remote-access thyroid surgery. Thyroid. 2016;**26**:331-337. DOI: 10.1089/thy.2015.0407

[7] Karakas E, Steinfeldt T, Gockel A, Schlosshauer T, Dietz C, Jäger J, et al. Transoral thyroid and parathyroid surgery–development of a new transoral technique. Surgery. 2011;**150**(1):108-115. DOI: 10.1016/j.surg.2010.12.016

[8] Anuwong A. Transoral endoscopic thyroidectomy vestibular approach: A series of the first 60 human cases. World Journal of Surgery. 2016;**40**:491-497. DOI: 10.1007/s00268-015-3320-1

[9] Sasanakietkul T, Jitpratoom P, Anuwong A. Transoral endoscopic parathyroidectomy vestibular approach: A novel scarless parathyroid surgery. Surgical Endoscopy. 2017;**31**:3755-3763. DOI: 10.1007/s00464-016-5397-5

[10] Chen H. Annals of Surgery;**236**(5):552-553

[11] Brennan MF, Doppman JL, Marx SJ, Spiegel AM, Brown EM, Aurbach GD. Reoperative parathyroid surgery for persistent hyperparathyroidism. Surgery. 1978;**83**(6):669-676

[12] Tibblin S, Bondeson A, Ljungberg O. Annals of Surgery. 1982;**195**(3):245-252

[13] Udelsman R. Six hundred fifty-six consecutive explorations for primary hyperparathyroidism. Annals of Surgery. 2002;**235**:665-670

[14] Udelsman R, Donovan PI, Sokoll LJ. One hundred consecutive minimally invasive parathyroid explorations. Annals of Surgery. 2000;**232**:331-339

[15] Bergenfelz A, Kanngiesser V, Zielke A, Nies C, Rothmund M. Conventional bilateral cervical exploration versus open minimally invasive parathyroidectomy under local anaesthesia for primary hyperparathyroidism. The British Journal of Surgery. 2005;**92**(2):190-197. DOI: 10.1002/bjs.4814

[16] Karakas E, Schneider R, Rothmund M, Bartsch DK, Schlosser K. Initial surgery for benign primary hyperparathyroidism: An analysis of 1,300 patients in a teaching hospital. World Journal of Surgery. 2014;**38**(8):2011-2018. DOI: 10.1007/s00268-014-2520-4